Eat Right for Life

How healthy foods can keep you living longer, stronger and disease-free

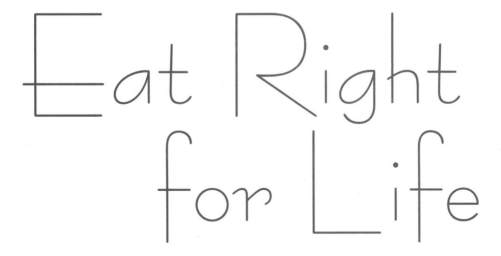

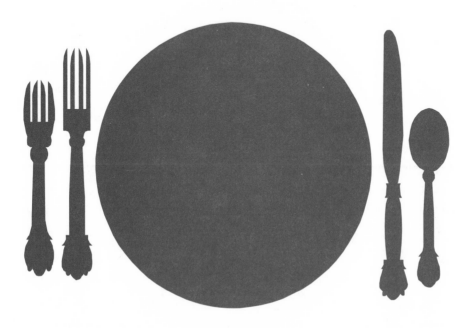

14   13   12   11   10   5   4   3   2   1

Library of Congress Control Number: 2010925821

ISBN-13: 978-1-4402-1132-4

ISBN-10: 1-4402-1132-9

Cover Design: Rachael Knier

Designed by: Joan Heiob Moyers

Edited by: Candy Wiza

Betterway Home a division of F+W Media, Inc.

4700 East Galbraith Rd.

Cincinnati, OH 45236

800-283-0963

www.betterwaybooks.com

BETTER WAY HOME

Distribúted in Canada by Fraser Direct
100 Armstrong Avenue
Georgetown, Ontario L7G 5S4
Canada

Distributed in Australia by Capricorn Link
P.O. Box 704
Windsor, NSW 2756
Australia

Distributed in the U.K. and Europe by
F+W Media International
Brunel House
Newton Abbot
Devon TQ12 4PU
England
Tel: (+44) 1626 323200
Fax: (+44) 1626 323319
E-mail: postmaster@davidandcharles.co.uk

Dedication

Casey Kellar, for inspiration and making this work possible.

Susan Salonisen, for her encouragement and knowledgeable suggestions.

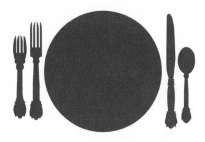

Acknowledgments

I wish to thank the following:
Susan Salonisen, for all of the recipes in this book.
The people of Kona, Hawaii who donated to
The Heart and Nutrition Foundation in 1985.

Contents

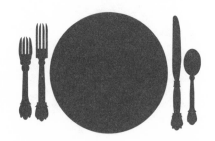

INTRODUCTION TO NUTRITIONAL
PHARMACOLOGY   7

chapter one

THE PHARMACY IN YOUR KITCHEN —
MOTHER NATURE KNOWS BEST
HEART DISEASE   11

The False Cholesterol Theory

The Copper Cure

Cause of Cardiovascular Deaths

Heart Failure Due to Lack of Oxygen

Copper: Critically Necessary for a Healthy Heart

Copper Deficency in Our Diet

Our Body's Copper Requirements

A Guide to Dietary Copper

Blackstrap Molasses: Your Heart's Greatest Friend

CANCER - P. 18

Cancer Theories and Studies

Causes of Cancer

Inadequate Cancer Theories

Cancer and Non-Industrialized Countries

Oxygen and Enzymes

The Fundamental Cause of Cancer

Effects of Copper Compounds on Tumors

Cancer Treatment

Chemotherapy: Is It Useless?

Curing Cancer

Prevent Cancer, Just by Eating!

Benefits of Selenium

Alternative Therapies for Cancer

ARTHRITIS - P. 31

Dr. Schep is a Human Study

Toss the Pain Relievers

Studies of Omega-3 Supplementation

Incorporate Omega-3 Fatty Acids

The Omega-6 and Omega-3 Ratio in the Diet

Krill Oil

Our Recommended Supplements

Restoration Through Nutrients

Strengthen Your Ligaments

Work It Out

Plantar Fasciitis

GLUTEN ALLERGIES - P. 48

Grain Family Relationships

Foods Containing Gluten

Grains and Flours for a Gluten-Free Lifestyle

Vitamin A to the Rescue

Gluten-Free Foods

chapter two

CHANGE YOUR LIFESTYLE AND
DITCH THE DIETS   53

"Big Food": The Processed Food Industry

Weight Control

Protein Is a Super Food

The Truth and Secrets About Weight Loss

The Cholesterol Myth

The Diet Summary

chapter three

WHAT CAN WE EAT?   81

Well-Balanced Variety is Key

Copper in the Diet

Omega-3 and Omega-9

Vitamin C

Anti-oxidants

Protein

Probiotics

Fiber

Food Substitutions

chapter four

WHY RAW IS BETTER   88

What Is Eating Raw?

Heat and What It Does to Our Food

Raw Food Facts

Raw Food and Your Thyroid

Making the Most of Meat

Cruciferous Vegetables

Beef Jerky

Raw Milk

Pastuerization

Organic Milk

chapter five

NATURE KNOWS BETTER THAN THE
FOOD MANUFACTURERS   99

The Nutrition Label

Fat Calories

Daily Value Percentages

The Salt Story

Label Claims: What They Really Mean

chapter six

A HEALTHY COLON –
A HEALTHY BODY   105

Digestive Health

Foods for Better Bowel Health

chapter seven

SO, YOU HAVE A SWEET TOOTH?   110

Infectious Diseases

Infection-Fighting White Blood Cells

The Lack and Benefits of Vitamin C

Sugar - The Sad Truth About the Sweet Treat

Sugar Alternatives

chapter eight

AIR, WATER AND EXERCISE AIR   117

Tune Up Your Lungs for the Indy 500 of Life

Poor Breathing Effects

Proper At-Rest Breathing Techniques

Water and our Body

Dehydration

Types of Water: Good and Bad

Excercise

chapter nine

100 BEST FOODS TO CURE DISEASE
AND MAINTAIN A HEALTHY MIND
AND BODY   125

Our Top 100 Recommend Foods – A to Z

chapter ten

RECIPES FOR HEALTHY, DISEASE-FREE
LIVING AND THEIR BENEFITS   168

Heart-Healthy Recipes

Fiber-Rich Recipes

Recipes Using Natural Sweeteners

Raw Food Recipes

Gluten-Free Recipes

BIBLIOGRAPHY   217

INDEX   221

TABLES   224

GLOSSARY   229

ABOUT THE AUTHORS   238

Introduction to Nutritional Pharmacology

Want to look fabulous, feel healthy and vibrant, and be immune to cancer and heart disease? Go back to basics! All of the vitamins, minerals, and nutrients you need to be healthy, strong, and gorgeous can be found in fresh foods. Think of how lean and strong our ancestors were and how obesity and the wide range of diseases we fight didn't rear their heads until processed, refined, packaged foods went mass market. Coincidence? Not by a long shot.

You'll even find the same effects in domestic animals because of their consumption of highly processed, refined foods. Wild animals in their natural habitats are muscular, energetic, and efficient meal planners. Animals kept as pets tend to be more overweight, under exercised, and have more of a tendency to succumb to illnesses that are not found in wild animals. This is because nature didn't intend for animals to eat from a bag or can — and neither were we!

From the beginning of time, all animals (and later humans) received their nutrients, vitamins, minerals and other essential supplements from vegetation. Even carnivores when preying on herbivores eat bodies that are saturated with essential vital nutrients from plants.

As time passes and plants and animals continue to grow and evolve, species relationships have been formed that benefit both plants and animals. That is, the plants benefit the animals, and the animals benefit from the plants. While these relationships are purely instinctual, they are extremely efficient and beneficial.

The result over millions of years from this co-evolution between plants and animals is extremely important to our health. Over time, the plants that made the animals the healthiest have had their seeds scattered or pollinated the most. This has resulted in plants, worldwide, having the potential to cure all disease. Today, we respond the best to cures using plants and herbs that have been used for millions of years while not responding well to synthetic drugs that have only been around for a hundred years or less.

more prevalent than ever. Nature, with its millions of years experience, produces what doctors have only practiced for 100 years.

Our bodies always will react better to natural remedies than synthetic drugs, which can cause severe, damaging side effects, and often are prescribed inaccurately.

Because our bodies were made to eat natural foods, they are not programmed to respond to or process synthetic medicines. Current day studies and experiments show that the human body happily accepts and uses natural drugs, or drugs that have been made with organic ingredients (plants, fruits, vegetables, etc.), and that synthetic drugs can be less effective and cause severe side effects.

Synthetic medicines generally contain only one active ingredient and do not contain additives to offset or counteract the side effects associated with the active ingredient. Medicines made from plants, however, tend to contain several active ingredients extracted from one plant (or plants) in the same family, that work together to balance or counteract possible side effects.

In Germany, the government has produced official monographs (as many as 181) indicating which plant drugs can be sold by pharmacies and what cures the marketer is allowed to claim for each plant drug. There even are monographs on plants that are used

Animal Pharmacology Facts

BISON: Roaming bison fed on grass fields, cropping the grass and then moving on. Later, the bison returned to the cropped fields to relieve themselves, thereby fertilizing the fields and allowing for fresh grass growth. After cropping and fertilizing one area, the bison would move on and repeat the process in another location. Once they cropped and fertilized the second location, they would return to the original location, which now had new growth to start the process over again.

MONKEYS: Monkeys thrive on foliage and wild fruits. They also are known for scattering or throwing the wild fruit seeds and pits after they are done consuming the fruits. The seeds grow and multiply, producing more fruit to be eaten and more seeds to be scattered. This natural behavior creates plenty of supply for the created demand. Interestingly, monkeys also use the forest as a pharmacy. Capuchin monkeys in Costa Rica rub themselves thoroughly with the leaves of the piper plant. Research has shown that the juice in the plant's leaves works as an insect repellent and wards off bacterial and fungus infections. And Colobus monkeys eat charcoal from the burned wood caused by forest fires. Some leafy plants in their diets contain cyanide and the charcoal absorbs the cyanide.

Over the past 100 years or so, modern medicine has made leaps and bounds and chemists have learned to make chemicals, synthetic prescription and over-the-counter medicines, but still, disease and obesity are for heart disease and reducing the size of cancerous tumors! These monographs mainly concentrate on European and some Middle Eastern plants and do not even begin to deal with the extensive knowledge about plants throughout the rest of the world.

You may be wondering how European monographs and recent studies make it possible for you to treat your ailments with plants. While we do not live in a forest or on a prairie, we do have fast-paced, busy lives and careers. But, we, too, can take advantage of the pharmacy in our kitchen to live and feel better. Keep reading and we will teach you how you can easily incorporate healthy, delicious, disease-fighting foods into your diet and your busy day.

Do you want to take that first step and learn how the foods you eat can help cure your ailments, make you look younger and help fight cancer? — You already have. The first step was picking up this book. Now, keep reading and we'll unlock the secrets to pain-free joints, younger-looking skin, a cancer and heart disease-free body and a trim figure by simply eating!

Mistletoe — it's not just for kissing! European mistletoe commonly is used to kill tumors!

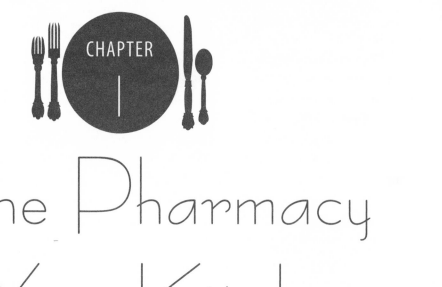

CHAPTER
1

The Pharmacy in Your Kitchen
– MOTHER NATURE KNOWS BEST

Do you ever feel rushed, out of time or unorganized? Do you sometimes forget to plan meals ahead of time so you grab drive-thru or pop a frozen pizza in the oven instead? Do you ever rely on prepackaged snacks or meals to get you through a hectic day? While these kinds of foods do help get you through the day — they are cutting years off of your life. These foods contain preservatives, gluten and high amounts of calories and fats. But more important is what these foods don't have. When our body does not get enough essential vitamins, nutrients, proteins and minerals, it starts to get weak. When the body is weak, disease creeps in. That's why it's important to give your body what it needs so it can stay strong, healthy, pain free and slim.

We have outlined some of the most serious diseases stemming from nutrient deficiencies as well as what to eat to prevent and/or fight off these serious diseases. We've also included a list of the top 100 cancer- and disease-fighting foods along with a description of why each food is a powerhouse of benefits. Use the precursory valuable information and enjoy the recipe section in Chapter 10 full of delicious, easy-to-prepare meals that will help you fight disease and Eat Right for Life!

HEART DISEASE

For the first time in the popular press, we now reveal that cholesterol has nothing to do with heart disease and show that the studies indicating this are completely flawed. It is a shortage of the trace mineral copper in our diets that is the true cause of heart disease.

Copper makes an enzyme called superoxide dismutase (SOD) that prevents plaque formation and arteries from closing and also makes veins and arteries stronger and more flexible. The USDA has done dozens of studies withholding copper from rats, mice, chickens and pigs and they immediately got heart attacks. (Believe it or not, there actually was one human study with the same result.) And the government full well knows this. Unfortunately, the U.S. diet contains very little copper compared to a natural diet because of factory-farming methods and harmful food-processing methods.

Unbeknownst to most people, heart disease is one of the most common and dangerous diseases in the United States. Every year, heart disease kills millions of people, approximately one death every minute in the United States. In our opinion, heart disease is the most serious health issue the United States currently is facing.

The information in this section is ground breaking, and you will not find it in any other book on nutrition or health, nor will you find it in medical journals or texts. It is being revealed for the first time in this book. At the end of this chapter, you will find our version of the Super Heart Diet — a diet rich in delicious, heart-healthy foods that will keep your heart strong and your taste buds happy.

Before we reveal the truth about heart disease, let's take a look at how heart disease currently is viewed. The present day theory concludes heart disease is caused by high cholesterol. Sadly, though, just as many people with low cholesterol die from heart disease as those with high cholesterol. Low cholesterol levels, while a good thing for your overall heath and well-being, will not exempt you from heart disease.

THE FALSE CHOLESTEROL THEORY

In 1963, researchers fed laboratory mice a diet consisting of 58 percent sugar, 28 percent lard, and a mineral saturated mixture. This combination was considered a high saturated fat diet called No. 2 USP XIII. These saturated fats occur in eggs, meat and milk, especially when animals are corn fed (as opposed to grass fed).

After nine weeks on the diet, arterial thrombosis (the formation of a blood clot inside a blood vessel, which obstructs the flow of blood through the circulatory system) began to occur. After 18 weeks, only a few mice were still alive.

Based upon this experiment, the medical community speculated that saturated fats increased cholesterol and fat, and that if too much cholesterol (a fat-like substance) was in your blood, it would build up in the walls of your arteries. Over time, the buildup causes "hardening of the arteries," (arteries become narrowed and blood flow to the heart is slowed or blocked). Blood carries oxygen to the heart, so if the arteries are narrowed or clogged, you may feel symptoms such as chest pain and light-headedness. If the blood supply to a portion of the heart is completely cut off by a blockage, the result is a heart attack.

However, another study, The Tecumseh

study[2], conducted from 1959 to 1979 (more information is available on the Internet), showed that saturated fat intake has no effect on cholesterol levels.

Now, we will explain why the lard in the mice's diets was not the cause of the thrombosis. One of the best examples is "Falling Disease," which has been observed in cattle.

THE COPPER CURE

In his book, "Trace Elements in Human and Animal Nutrition," Professor E.J. Underwood wrote that in the 1930s, Australian cattle were herded by riders on horseback and would sometimes collapse and die. It was observed, however, that this did not occur in areas near vineyards where grapes were sprayed with Bordeaux mixture, (a mixture of copper and lime). The soils in the areas where the cows were collapsing and dying was analyzed and found to be extremely deficient in copper.

At the time of the study, it was not known why the copper reduced the incidence of the disease. By chance, beginning in the 1950s and continuing through present day, further discoveries have been made concerning the effect of the trace mineral on our health.

In a study at the Utah College of Medicine[3], rats were deprived of copper. The copper was stripped from their diet by feeding them only dried whole milk powder with sugar and mineral supplements that excluded copper. The finding was that the

Lucille Ball ("I Love Lucy") and Jack Ritter ("Three's Company") both passed away due to aortic rupture. Jack Ritter's family actually sued the doctors who treated Mr. Ritter, for misdiagnosis. (See later reports on why our food lacks copper.)

offspring of the rats on the copper-deficient diet were unable to hold blood in their veins and arteries, forcing bleeding in the surrounding tissues.

In 1963, Carlton[4] fed 20 chickens a diet rich in all minerals except copper. Within 56 days, 16 of the 20 birds had died, nine of them from aortic rupture. Those are amazingly scary numbers!

CAUSE OF CARDIOVASCULAR DEATHS

Dr. Ralph Spiekerman[5] of the Mayo Clinic performed 1,326 autopsies in 1962 and found that the biggest cause of heart disease-related deaths (43 percent) was irregular heartbeat, or fibrillation. The second highest cause (39 percent) was due to death of the heart muscle from lack of blood flow and oxygen. This means that virtually all heart disease deaths are either from stoppage or lack of oxygen from poor circulation.

HEART FAILURE DUE TO LACK OF OXYGEN

The other major cause of cardiovascular death is lack of circulation. The body burns sugar and carbohydrates to provide energy and heat. Oxygen from the air is used to burn the carbohydrates, which produces heat and carbon dioxide.

One of the side effects of this process, is that a very, very, small portion of the oxygen produces a superoxide radical. A superoxide radical is an oxygen atom that is extremely reactive and damaging to the body, especially the arteries. (In laymen's terms, a superoxide radical can be visualized as a burning oxygen molecule.) This superoxide radical can damage arterial walls, which then sends a signal to the white blood cells to come and repair the damage, causing plaque to form (according to Dr. Judy Berliner of the

University of California, Los Angeles[6]). This causes inflammation and lack of circulation due to lack of blood flow, eventually causing the heart muscle to die.

Conventional wisdom blames lipoproteins, which the white blood cells bind to form or cause plaque. However, there is an enzyme in every single cell of the body that can hunt down this superoxide radical and destroy it. The technical name is superoxide dismutase (SOD). Can you guess what superoxide dismutase is made of? You guessed it — COPPER!

Studies[7] have shown that the higher the copper intake the more superoxide dismutase enzyme present in the body. Conversely, less copper in the body means less superoxide dismutase in the body.

Superoxide (not to be confused with superoxide dismutase) causes arteries to constrict, cutting off blood flow and plaque to form, causing inflammation in the arteries.

Superoxide dismutase destroys the superoxide. The following studies confirm the findings.

In 2005, Changdong Yan[8] noted that superoxide dismutase improves the function of arteries in mice causing improved circulation.

In 1999, Qiang Liu[9] reported that superoxide dismutase counteracts vasoconstriction caused by superoxide.

Sean Didion[10], showed superoxide dismutase prevents inflammation in the arteries, which reduces blood flow.

What does all of this mean in plain English? Copper addresses all the forms of heart disease!

Dr. Schep's finding concludes: The body normally and naturally protects the arteries by utilizing SOD (made from copper). Cut-

ting down on lipoproteins (LDL/HDL), as is the conventional wisdom, is not the way the body functions. Plaque will only form due to a deficiency in superoxide dismutase, caused by a deficiency of copper in the diet. So instead of trying to combat plaque and poor circulation, increase your copper!

COPPER: CRITICALLY NECESSARY FOR A HEALTHY HEART

The most dramatic and conclusive study supporting copper is that of Hill, Starcher and Kim, from the University of North Carolina at Raleigh[11]. In their ground-breaking work, they struck at the core of the cause of heart disease. Unfortunately, very few people are aware of their outstanding work. The information simply is not being shared with the public and/or medical students. Until now, no popular book on health contained this information. You are leaps and bounds ahead of the mass public in the race for good cardiovascular health and wellness!

When conducting their studies, Hill, Starcher and Kim already knew that the veins, arteries and cardiovascular tissue were mainly made of two proteins, namely collagen and elastin protein. They also knew that in the past researchers conducting similar studies always found the elastin tissue in copper-deficient animals to be defective. This resulted in aortic ruptures, aneurysms and problems with the elastin tissue, which provides flexibility to the arteries.

Then they analyzed the elastin tissue from chicks that were copper deficient and made an important discovery: The elastin had too much lysine in it. Lysine is an amino acid, or a protein-building block. Following, they did a study of the enzyme necessary to convert lysine to healthy elastin tissue and came to the startling discovery — the enzyme was a copper-containing enzyme. The truth became apparent: Without copper, this enzyme cannot be made by the body and the body cannot make elastin tissue, therefore, it cannot make healthy arteries

Drs. Leslie M. Klevay, and K.E. Viestenz[12] performed an experiment in 1982 in which they fed rats a copper-deficient diet. Seven out of the 10 rats developed abnormal cardiograms. The rats fed a copper-filled diet did not suffer the abnormal cardiograms. The average lifespan of the rats fed the diet lacking in copper was one third that of the rats that did not have the copper stripped out of their diets. They reincorporated copper into the diet of those rats who had developed the abnormal cardiograms and noticed marked improvement in the rats' cardiovascular health. Amazing!

In 1978, A. Swift[13] found copper to be a better prescription for treating arrhythmia than prescribed drugs called beta blockers. Beta blockers can have severe, detrimental side effects and, copper, acting as a beta blocker, is an all-natural nutrient that has no side effects.

Earlier we discussed the sugar/lard diet (No. 2 USP XIII), which researchers claimed was proof that cholesterol causes heart disease. Researching further, Dr. L. M. Klevay[14] repeated the experiment in 1984 and found, yes, the mice got atherosclerosis. But then he pointed out that the diet did not contain copper. In a new experiment using mice, Kelvay added copper to their drinking water and they did not get atherosclerosis! This conclusively disproves the cholesterol theory and shows that copper deficiency causes heart disease.

COPPER DEFICIENCY IN OUR DIET

As time goes on, lower and lower levels of copper are being found in our food. This most likely is due to the mineral being depleted from our soils by the use of the same agricultural lands over and over every year, without properly replacing the copper and other nutrients (such as iron and zinc) that are removed by the plants being harvested.

According to Leslie M. Klevay[15], a 1976 article in Nutritional Reports International reported that in 1942 bananas had 2.1 parts per million (ppm) of copper (2.1 milligrams per kilogram or 2 pounds). In 1966, bananas had 0.66 ppm. During that same period, egg yolks went from 4 ppm to 2.4 ppm; white bread from 3.4 ppm to 0.19 ppm. Only egg whites went up; 0.3 ppm to 1.7 ppm. But even at that level, egg whites are not a good source of copper. During this time period (1942-1966) there was a *44 percent increase* in the death rate due to heart disease and fat consumption actually decreased.

OUR BODY'S COPPER REQUIREMENTS

The recommended daily allowance of copper in the human diet has been set at 2 ppm. Our criticism is that this is the minimum amount required to prevent deficiency symptoms in most people and it is not the optimum amount required for best health.

In the Journal of Food Science (1960), C. F. Mills[16] states that 10 ppm of copper is necessary for melanin (the dark color in skin and hair) formation in rats. Three ppm is required for growth, and 1 ppm was found necessary for the formation of hemoglobulin. It appears that gray hair may appear in humans even with copper levels just below 10 ppm. All the severe deficiency symptoms in chickens, mice and rats were caused at a copper intake range of 0.7 ppm to 0.9 ppm.

In a 1986 copy of Lab Animal Science[17], Dr. W. Stephen Damron and Dr. A. R. Menino, Jr. reported that they gave pregnant mice copper in the range of 1 ppm to 11 ppm. The doctors reported that at 1 ppm, embryos failed to develop. At 3 ppm, embryos showed a lower rate of development. At the 4 ppm to 11 ppm copper range, embryo development was greater. The apparent conclusion for pregnant mice, is that they need 4 ppm or more of copper for normal pregnancy and that even 11 ppm is okay.

Dr. Schep was teaching Dr. Damron's class at the time the paper was being written and he was able to help proofread the manuscript. The findings spurred him to do further literature research, where he was able to discover all the works that had been published on the importance of copper for the heart.

Since the astounding effects of copper have not been widely advertised, it was hard to find a copper experiment performed using people, instead of animals. However, we did find one very interesting experiment.

S. Riser[18] of the U.S. Department of Agriculture outlined a study he performed to help determine if fructose, a form of refined sugar, lowered copper levels in the body more than just starch. His subjects ranged in age from 21 to 57 and they were fed a diet containing 1 milligram of copper per day. Unfortunately, the study had to be terminated three weeks early due to four of the subjects developing heart problems during the study. One subject even had a heart attack! This resulted because the proper research had not been conducted prior to the study. You see, giving a fructose-high diet to people, especially men over age 40, who have low copper intake, is extremely dangerous, as proved by the reaction of the subjects.

Unfortunately, the Internet is extremely misinformed about copper. The popular view is that it is a heavy metal and toxic. Therefore, criticism of the findings in this book may be almost automatic.

Some critics argue that oysters, clams and mussels contain not only copper and zinc, which are beneficial, but also mercury, lead and cadmium, which are not, and encourage people to avoid those foods. One Web site warns not to exceed 1 milligram of copper per day because you may get Wilson's disease. Wilson's disease is a genetic defect of copper metabolism, allowing copper to build up in the body. The prevalence of Wilson's disease, a rare disease, is one in 30,000 people. So adjusting your copper intake to below one milligram per day because of a fear of Wilson's disease or lead, mercury or cadmium poisoning simply is ridiculous. It's also entirely misleading in light of the overwhelming scientific studies of copper intake in laboratory animals. Consider this: Mayo Clinic surgeon Dr. Spiekerman found that if you take anyone over the age of 30, no matter what the cause of death upon autopsy, you will find symptoms of cardiovascular disease in three out of four of those bodies. This means that Americans, as a general rule, do not have healthy hearts.

Statistics show that you are at a much greater risk of dying of heart disease than of mercury, lead and/or cadmium poisoning. We do not hear of any persons dying of mercury or cadmium poisoning, especially from the small exposure you would get from incorporating healthy amounts of these foods into your regular diet. However, we regularly hear of friends losing someone in their family due to heart attacks and have many friends who are under care for heart disease. In addition, we'll discuss later adequate intake of Vitamin C and how it can protect you against heavy metal poisoning.

We challenge anyone, who would argue that copper is a toxic and heavy metal or that we should not have an intake of more than 1 milligram per day in our food, to show us one scientific study proving their theory.

FOOD	PPM
WHITE SUGAR	0.2 to 0.6
MILK PRODUCTS	0.1 to 0.9
BEEF (MUSCLE MEATS)	0.4 to 0.8
VEGETABLES	0.5 to 1.5
REFINED GRAINS	1.3 to 1.9
UNREFINED GRAINS	2.4 to 3.6
DRIED BEANS & PEAS	6.5 to 10.0
NUTS	6.0 to 15.0
BLACKSTRAP MOLASSES	15.0 to 20.0
LIVER	22.0 to 30.0
OYSTERS	25.0 to 31.0
UN-HULLED SESAME SEEDS	40.0 to 41.0

A GUIDE TO DIETARY COPPER

The copper content of heart muscle decreases with age[19]. Therefore, why would it be surprising that men over 40 and women after menopause have increased rates of heart disease? An expectant mother must supply 0.34 milligrams of copper to her unborn baby every day[20], a tough act to follow on an average American intake of 1.0 milligram a day. So, if you are pregnant, yes, oysters, bitter chocolate and cashew nuts are definitely okay! And if you are over 40, you must make a deliberate effort to increase your intake of copper. (Dr. Schep takes 4 milligrams a day.)

At left is a rough guide to copper levels in common foods.

It's amazing that the high levels of rampant heart disease haven't sky rocketed to more astounding levels. If your diet consists solely of white sugar, dairy, meat, vegetables and refined grains, your average copper intake will be 0.7 milligram per kilogram of food per day (a kilogram is 2.2 lbs).

The average American may have a daily menu similar to this:

BREAKFAST
French toast, syrup, margarine, milk
    or
Apple juice, corn flakes, white toast with margarine, milk
    or
Coffee cake, margarine, applesauce, milk

LUNCH
Vegetable beef stew, white roll, margarine, vanilla ice cream, strawberry jelly
    or
Barbecue chicken, salad, French dressing, cheddar cheese bread, margarine, shortbread cookies
    or
Crispy chicken, steamed rice, broccoli, white

bread, grape jelly

DINNER

Orange juice, grilled chicken, noodle casserole, steamed vegetables

or

Minestrone soup, potatoes, corn bread, butter

or

Grilled beef, French fries, carrots, vanilla pudding

SNACKS

Chips, flavored coffee drinks, pretzels

or

Cookies, soda, prepackaged jerky

or

Candy, energy drink, popcorn

Such a diet only supplies 0.7 milligrams of copper per day, a number that has been shown to cause severe heart disease in animals! This may come as surprise to most folks. Just as surprising — this diet is similar to what you get in a hospital cardiovascular ward!

Why is our diet so lacking in copper? Here are a few reasons:

Lack of nuts.

White bread instead of whole-wheat bread.

Polished rice instead of brown rice.

Refined sugar.

No legumes.

No liver or other organ meats.

Little or no shellfish, such as oysters.

We can confidently predict that if you begin to incorporate beans, peas, nuts, liver and/or oysters in your daily diet, you will not suffer from heart disease — no matter how many eggs or how much meat you eat.

So, how do we get 2 milligrams of copper? The easiest way is to consume some of the following:

4 ounces walnuts or almonds.

6 ounces peanuts (peanuts have the lowest copper level of all nuts).

8 ounces dried beans (beans weigh more after they are cooked – be sure to weigh dry beans).

3 ounces liver (or Braunschweiger – liverwurst sausage).

3 ounces oysters.

3.5 ounces cashew nuts.

Need some creative ways to incorporate those ingredients into your diet? Try these easy, delicious options:

Add chopped walnuts or slivered almonds to a fresh green salad with sliced apples and grated cheese.

Add four ounces of beans to a wrap at lunch or toss four ounces into your soup or salad at dinner.

Make a three-bean chili or soup for dinner and enjoy leftovers for lunch the next day — easy, affordable and delicious!

Make liver and onions for dinner. This doesn't have to be your grandma's dry, chewy liver recipe. Try a delicious rub made from fresh ingredients, and check out the book "Quick-Fix Healthy Mix: 225 healthy and affordable recipes to stock your kitchen," for healthy, inexpensive sauces and seasonings.

Coat oysters in cracker crumbs, salt and pepper and bake for a delicious, crispy treat.

Serve oysters with steamed asparagus — a healthy, filling and delicious meal.

Snack on chopped mixed nuts (cashews,

almonds, brazils, peanuts). with red raisins.

You should be getting the balance of copper from your normal diet (0.7 to 1 milligrams) on the condition that you eliminate white sugar. White sugar contains no copper, yet increases the body's need for copper. And eat whole grains, not refined grains such as white flour and polished rice.

BLACKSTRAP MOLASSES: YOUR HEART'S GREATEST FRIEND

Experimentation with white sugar, which contains less than 0.2 milligrams of copper, has shown that when mixed into a diet made out of milk powder (when all other minerals except copper are supplemented) it causes devastating cardiovascular disease in lab animals (Klevay1981[14]).

When crude sugar from the sugar cane is processed, the sugar is refined to make it as pure as possible. The dark material is rejected and considered a waste product. However, that "waste" actually is an amazing, well-kept secret called *blackstrap molasses*.

Blackstrap molasses contains all of the copper that originally was present in the sugar cane sap. Since most of the water has been removed, the copper, zinc, iron and other minerals are in concentrated levels, making it not only tasty but extremely good for protecting your heart.

The molasses has a copper content between 15 ppm to 20 ppm, depending on the copper levels in the soil where the sugar cane was harvested. This level is about the same or a little higher than three ounces of almonds, which roughly contains 15 ppm of copper. But the copper level is not quite as high as oysters or liver, which register approximately 25 or 30 ppm. However, it's very easy to add into your daily diet. Try these simple ways to add heart-healthy copper-filled blackstrap molasses into your daily diet:

Stir molasses in warm milk, tea or coffee.

Mix one part blackstrap molasses with two parts maple syrup.

Add warm milk and blackstrap molasses to your oatmeal for a healthy, yummy breakfast.

Add a healthy twist to traditional homemade cookies (look online for great recipes).

Bake homemade healthy and delicious whole-grain bread with blackstrap molasses.

CANCER

Sadly, cancer currently is the biggest cause of mortality, after heart disease, causing about 13 percent of human deaths.

In countries where natural village holistic agriculture is carried out, there is no cancer and, yet, Americans have a high rate of cancer. Why is this happening and what is the cause? Keep reading as we show you a radical new discovery supported by dozens of scientific papers never before reported in popular literature to help you understand.

All cancerous cells have low levels of copper and copper is part of an enzyme called superoxide dismutase (SOD), which protects the cell against toxins. Chemotherapy, surgery and radiation therapy do not address the cause of cancer — a copper deficiency — and therefore do not cure

According to the American Cancer Society, 7.6 million people died from cancer in 2007.

cancer.

The stunning fact: The very toxins that cause cancer in cells are used in chemotherapy to attempt to kill the cells. There are many reports of natural therapies that are much more effective than chemotherapy and these therapies work by using anti-oxidants from fresh fruits, plants and vegetables to protect the cell against toxins. And although these are also recommended, copper is the most effective. We'll show you how to change your diet to get adequate copper and anti-oxidants (vitamin A, vitamin C, vitamin E and numerous other plant anti-oxidants into your diet).

When low levels of SOD in cancer cells are restored by adding copper — cancer cells become normal again!

CANCER THEORIES AND STUDIES

The current theories and accepted viewpoints on cancer are quite different than what the actual facts and studies show to be the true causes and prevention of cancer. You will find out that the common views concerning cancer may very well be inaccurate. And we'll report the true cause of cancer and how to combat it, something that has never been published in popular literature — until now!

The true cause of cancer is in complete agreement with the facts concerning the behavior of cancer. For example, in regions where people consume specific diets that are rich in the nutrients our body's cells need, serious illnesses (such as cancer) very rarely occur.

Civilized diets fail to provide the correct nutrition. Without sufficient amounts of nutrients from the food we eat, our cells cannot function normally and the lack of nutrients promotes abnormal cell growth and mutation. This is called cancer.

When abnormal cells are supplemented with the right amount of nutrients, *they can and will revert into normally functioning, healthy cells.*

Want to know how to easily incorporate sufficient nutrients to stave off cancer into your daily diet? We'll show you how with some easy, delicious, nutritious ways to live a cleaner, healthier lifestyle.

CAUSES OF CANCER

Cancer affects people of every nationality, gender, age group and region, even domestic animals are susceptible to cancer. While cancer does affect every age group, the risk of developing cancer does increase with age.

Cells become cancerous because they are not protected against free radicals due to an industrialized processed-food diet, which increases our free-radical load. The problem with a processed food diet? It's high in sugar, and low in copper and anti-oxidants, and all these increase our free radical load.

The trace element copper, missing in our diets, is the first defense against free-radical damage to the cell because it makes an enzyme called superoxide dismutase (SOD) in the cell; low levels of selenium and manganese also contribute to this defense. Anti-oxidants also make a huge important contribution to our defenses against cancer-causing free-radical damage, and we easily can add these into our diets with fruits and vegetables.

Cancer occurs in groups of cells that display uncontrolled growth (the splitting of cells when the body doesn't need to produce new cells, which creates a tumor) and invasion of surrounding tissues. Sometimes

---

Metastasize is the medical theory that doctors use to try and explain why cancer continues in the body after surgical or radiation removal of tumors. In this book, we show that cancer is caused by a lack of antioxidants in the diet, which affects the entire body. This means that the entire body is still susceptible to cancer after surgery, radiation or chemotherapy because the cause of the cancer has not been addressed. Therefore, the cancer can continue in any part of the body.

---

these growths spread to other locations of the body by travelling through the blood stream or lymph nodes. These three malignant properties of cancers differentiate them from benign tumors, which are limited to a specific area and do not invade neighboring cells or tissues and do not metastasize.

Most cancers do form a tumor or polyp, but other types of cancer, leukemia for instance, do not.

INADEQUATE CANCER THEORIES

Science is a beautiful thing. The scientific community is always able to come up with scenarios and corresponding theories. However, the dangerous thing about science is that while many theories exist, most often the theories are claimed to be or, understood to be, proven facts, even amongst prominent scientists, doctors and pharmacologists. Unfortunately, when these theories are confronted or challenged, the tendency is that the challenger is made to seem misspoken or uninformed to save face for the well-financed research projects or pharmaceutical companies.

According to Dr. John Boyd from The Center for the Biology of Chronic Disease (CBCD), in an article currently on the Internet, the ingrained policy of the National Institutes of Health (NIH) is that cancer is caused by a mutation to our genes and/or cells as a result of exposure to carcinogens. A carcinogen is defined as a chemical that can alter our genes and cells. As a result of the ability to change and/or alter our genes and cells, they mutate to produce tumors which result in cancer. However, in a study held in the United States of 180,000 cases of breast cancer, only 5 percent of patients had mutated genes. (Also see R.J. Jariwalla[21].)

This information sends mixed signals and is confusing to the masses to say the least. Dr. Boyd says the NIH is alleging that the cause of cancer is mutated genes and/or cells brought on by ingesting carcinogens. If that is true, how could it be possible that 9,000 women in the study had no mutated cells or genes? It could be true that one of the causes of cancer is mutated cells caused by carcinogens, but it obviously is not the only cause of cancer. So, why are the NIH, biotech companies and pharmaceutical companies investing billions of dollars in continued research on the "cause" of cancer (carcinogens) and not investing that money on finding the other, very real causes of cancer?

Another theory by Dr. Hannan Polansky[22] on the cause of cancer is that cancer is caused by viruses that enter the body's cells and interfere with our cell's mechanisms, causing them to become cancerous. The problem we find with this theory is that viruses are contagious and can spread from person to person, region to region and country to country within a matter of days. For instance, during the writing of this book, the Swine Flu was declared a pandemic. However, in countries such as Sri Lanka, breast and prostate cancer are almost non-existent and have been for as long as we have known. However, viruses and other communicable diseases are quite commonly spread. In addition, if the United States has a "cancer virus epidemic or pandemic," how is it possible that persons caring for cancer patients in the United States and other countries with higher cancer rates (as well as residents of countries like Sri Lanka where cancer has never existed), aren't experiencing dramatic increases in cancer?

Alternatively, is it possible that the immune systems of Americans may not be able to defeat the "virus," whereas the diet the Sinhalese eat provides them with the nutrients to boost their immune systems and fight off the virus? In either scenario, due to the extreme lack of breast and prostate cancer in Sri Lanka, as well as the fact that cancer is a non-communicable disease, we can be assured that breast and prostate can-

cer at least are not caused by a virus.

Another common theory is that estrogen causes breast cancer and testosterone causes prostate cancer. The belief is that women who take estrogen for menopause suffer increased contraction of cancer, and men who take testosterone to counteract the effects of aging show an increased contraction rate of prostate cancer.

This theory actually is in conflict with the proven facts:

Men have the highest level of testosterone in their bodies around the age of 30. Prostate cancer is proven to be almost unheard of at this young age. Testosterone levels start declining around age 45, almost exactly the same age when prostate cancer starts to creep into the scene.

Girls beginning puberty (pre-teen and early teen years) experience massive increases in estrogen levels with almost no occurrences of breast cancer in teen girls. However, during the beginning stages of menopause, estrogen levels begin rapidly decreasing and breast cancer rates start in-

Cancer Mortality per 100,000 persons (1996)

Type Of Cancer	UNITED STATES Male	Female	SRI LANKA Male	Female
COLON	19	19	0	0
LUNG	72	42	2	0
PROSTATE	28	N/A	2	N/A
BREAST	N/A	32	N/A	2
LUNG (including trachea and bronchus)	72	43	2	0
TOTALS	191	136	4	2

Source: World Health Statistics Annual (1996) World Health Organization.

creasing as women age and experience lowering levels of estrogen.

Many other published theories for the cause of cancer exist, including: using deodorants, cellular telephones and toothpaste; ingesting or using chlorinated water; using tobacco; wearing brassieres (yes, seriously); spending too much time in the sun; undergoing X-rays; and ingesting radon gas that

Tips for Growing a Healthy, Natural Garden Indoors

Purchase quality seeds. You get what you pay for and discount seeds may not have a great success rate.

Look for non-hybrid seeds. The added flair can be great, but hybrid seeds don't always offer the best tasting end product.

Use organic potting soil that is specifically marked for indoor use. Organic potting soil is rich in nutrients, vitamins and minerals and will produce a healthy fruit, vegetable or herb.

In the fall, winter, and early spring your plants will need extra light. A grow light or an inexpensive fluorescent light tube (30 to 50 watt bulbs) will give your plants just the right amount of light and warmth.

Lightly water your garden daily or every other day.

is released from the ground in the basement of your home. All of these theories have been funded with extraordinary amounts of money for research while the real causes of cancer, which we will get to next, are swept aside.

So, are you ready to get the real facts on how cancer is developed, how it can be fought, and how to protect yourself by simply eating? Let's get started!

CANCER AND NON-INDUSTRIALIZED COUNTRIES

First, take a look at the table on page 21 outlining the differences in the cancer mortality rates between males and females in the United States and Sri Lanka. This table is an excerpt from a publication in 1996 by the World Health Organization (WHO).

What stands out the most from the table is that for every 100,000 people in 1996, 32 women in the United States died from breast cancer and 28 men in the United States died from prostate cancer due to the American way of life. Fatty fast foods, nutrient-deficient meals, and over processed and preserved snacks and beverages play a huge part in this equation. Sinhalese do not have the availability or accessibility to the bad foods we Americans consume on a daily basis. In the same time period, only two Sri Lankan women died from breast cancer and only two Sri Lankan men died from prostate cancer. Coincidence? Not a chance.

So what exactly are Americans doing so differently than Sinhalese? The most crucial difference is that over three-quarters of the population of Sri Lanka grow their own food by using traditional farming methods that actually recycle vital soil nutrients and minerals back into the ground by fertilizing the soil with unused or decomposing foods and/or animal waste (manure). Sinhalese fertilizer consists of compost, manure, ash and silt, making it rich in over 72 trace elements and minerals. This means that the harvested crops are mineral and nutrient rich and the soil is not stripped or depleted, as they tend to be in America. The reason for this is that there are no modern and mechanized systems of farming, meaning less wear and tear on the soil as well as no use of petroleum-derived fertilizers that are unnatural and unhealthy for our bodies and our environment. U.S. fertilizer consists of petro-chemically derived fertilizer, acid purified rock phosphate and highly purified potassium and it is totally devoid of trace elements or minerals. Not stuff we want in our bodies, but stuff we are unknowingly ingesting on a daily basis.

Another amazing discovery we found during our research for this book — the cause of heart disease and the cause of cancer are the exact same thing – lack of copper! Copper is the "queen" of trace minerals and plays many vital roles in the body, including, but not limited to: reduces tissue damage caused by free radicals; assists in the development of body pigment called melanin; regulates thyroid functions; and helps the body absorb and utilize iron. How did America become copper deficient? We introduced petrochemicals, artificial sweeteners, unnatural preservatives, partially hydrogenated oils and trans fats into our daily routines. So how do we undo the damage we have inflicted upon ourselves? GO NATURAL! Grow your own fruits and vegetables, cut out quick foods with deadly ingredients and purchase organic products whenever possible.

You may be wondering how you are going to add natural farming or gardening to your schedule in addition to work, family, friends, children and everything else your busy lifestyle throws at you. Don't worry. We don't expect you to turn your backyard, balcony or window box into rice paddies or miniature farms. However, we will show you how to easily and economically replace the over processed, chemically enhanced foods with fresh, all-natural, mineral-rich foods from the comfort of your home or local grocery store.

OXYGEN AND ENZYMES

At the University of California, Los Angeles (UCLA), there is an amazing, five-story building called the Biomedical Library. The way to the library can be a little daunting; walls covered in portraits of past medical school deans; a huge botanical garden; and halls teeming with interns proudly displaying their stethoscopes. Once inside the library building, you can't help but feel impressed, as almost every medical journal, book, article and publication ever written by man is there. The section on cancer on the fifth floor is enormous and the selections are widely varied by type of cancer, theory, author and other distinguishing factors. These proudly displayed books certainly are not what we came for.

The book we are looking for, the book that comes the closest to outlining the true causes of cancer, is tucked away on a dark shelf in the corner close to the floor. The book is called Pathology of Oxygen[23], and was published in 1982. Chapter 13, our favorite, is written by several authors, one of which is Dr. John Sorenson of the University of Arkansas, Little Rock. Chapter 13 explains the difference of chemical composition between a healthy cell and a cancerous cell. The remarkable facts in this little book, which was hidden away, have remained virtually unknown since 1982, until now.

Chapter 13 explains that in all cells of air-breathing animals (animals that rely on oxygen for life), there is an enzyme called superoxide dismutase. This enzyme is not present in the cells of species not needing oxygen, like anaerobic bacteria or other bacteria.

Air-breathing cells, like ours, follow this process:

Take in oxygen.

Take in glucose or fats.

Use oxygen to burn glucose or fat to create energy; then,

Expel carbon dioxide.

Carbon can easily be used to make energy by burning it in oxygen. The problem is that we have to generate very high temperatures for this to happen. The extremely high temperature converts oxygen into a superoxide, giving it the energy to combine with the carbon to make carbon dioxide and heat.

In order for this process to work at body temperature, cells have to convert oxygen into superoxide. Superoxide is highly reactive and has the power to combine with the carbon and hydrogen contained in the glucose and fats we consume to convert them into heat, energy, carbon dioxide and water.

In simpler terms, this process is: breathe; eat; exercise; then dispel waste.

Superoxide is so reactive that any stray superoxide that comes into contact with the cell causes damage unless the cell is protected. If left unprotected, the damaged cell will work overtime to protect itself, causing it to multiply, break apart and become abnormal. These abnormal cells become cancerous tumors.

The body is much like the engine of a car. The combustion of gas (fuel) with air provides the energy to run the car. This process produces so much heat that if the engine is not cooled, it will become overheated and start to malfunction. In cars, a water-cooled radiator is installed to remove the heat and protect the engine.

In the body, *superoxide dismutase (SOD)* in the cells protects them against superoxide, which although necessary for life, can cause severe damage to cells.

There are a couple of different kinds of superoxide dismutase found in the body's cells. The most common is copper zinc superoxide dismutase, which we will call *Cu-Zn SOD* and the other is called manganese superoxide dismutase, which we will call *Mn SOD*. *Mn SOD* is found inside the mitochondria of the lungs of the cell where fuel is being burned to produce energy. *Cu-Zn SOD* is found in the fluid within the cell and gives the cell strong protection.

What does this mean in plain English? If the body does not get enough copper or manganese through the foods we eat, it cannot produce superoxide dismutase. Without superoxide dismutase, your cells can't protect themselves, and you, against harmful elements.

THE FUNDAMENTAL CAUSE OF CANCER

"Pathology of Oxygen" points out the one fact that is missing in all those other, highly esteemed books. Cancer cells are *cells that are deficient in Cu-Zn SOD and Mn SOD.* As a matter of fact, some cancer cells have been found to have no *Mn SOD* in them at all. Normal, healthy cells do not lack *Cu-Zn SOD and Mn SOD.* It is possible then, that cells turn cancerous because they have no protection against superoxide.

Also found in the UCLA Biomedical Library is a book titled "Progress in Medicinal Chemistry,"Vol. 26 (1989). In this book, there is an article written by Dr. John Sorensen that references no less than 24 published works by scientists who found that they could slow down tumor growth and increase survival of mice by using copper compounds that have similar activity to *Cu-Zn SOD*.

Another amazing piece of work is a 1979 thesis by a scientist named S. K. Sahu[24]. In his thesis he states: "Copper complex added to neuroblastoma culture medium caused differentiation of these neoplastic cells to normal neuronal cells in a concentration related manner." Translation: We took endocrine cancer cells, grew them in the lab and then treated them with a copper compound. They became normal cells. The effect increases when more copper compound is used.

EFFECTS OF COPPER COMPOUNDS ON TUMORS

In studies contained in "Pathology of Oxygen," the authors discuss a report on an experiment using mice. Tumors were induced in mice. The tumors were then injected with copper compounds with superoxide dismutase activity. After 22 days, the size of the tumors in the legs of mice not injected with SOD compounds had grown to 2.2 centimeters in size. In the tumors injected with SOD activity, each tumor was, on the average, 1 centimeter or less.

In another experiment by Dr. Petkau in 1997, tumors in mice were injected with *Cu-Zn SOD*. Despite the fact that only one injection to each tumor was given, the treated tumors grew more slowly than the untreated tumors for 40 days. From day 41 to day 56, the growth rate decreased even

further. (See also Larry Ob[...] ed Cu-Zn SOD to increase[...] mals.) The normal, natural w[...] Cu-Zn SOD by *increasing co*[...]

CANCER TREATMENT

We have been listening to the politicians debating health care on the radio. Unfortunately, in our opinion, the ancient Greek philosopher's statement that rulers have a block of wood for heads, still remains true. These politicians are convinced that if someone is diagnosed with cancer, and denied chemotherapy or surgery because of affordability, it would be a death sentence. Therefore you and I should pay for their ineffective synthetic drug treatment by socialized health care.

Death sentence? We don't think so.

CHEMOTHERAPY: IS IT USELESS?

There are a growing number of authorities stating that chemotherapy and surgery are useless. And we have decided to bring to your attention at least one (of many) studies showing it is useless. It is a comprehensive study by Drs. Morgan, Ward and Baton, "Clinical Oncology" (2004) 16: 549-560. At the time of writing this book, it also is published on the Internet. The background of the publication is that all persons diagnosed with cancer have a mean (average) survival rate; defined as the time after diagnosis when 50 percent of the persons are still alive. For pancreatic cancer, this has been reported to be one to two years, for breast cancer this is reported to be 20 years (Dr. Harriet Denz-Penhey, Western University, Crawley Australia). These doctors used the measurement to gauge how many people were still alive years after being diagnosed with cancer. The average number is somewhere around 60 percent.

Then, they studied 10,661 people and determined what the rate of survivability was for persons that had chemotherapy versus those that did not have chemotherapy. Are you ready for this? They found that only 2 percent more people survived five years or more after chemotherapy than those who did not! This 2 percent probably is not significant and within measurement error. The conclusion: If you have chemotherapy treatment, you will not live any longer than if you do not have chemotherapy.

After the report came to light, the Australian doctors were immediately interviewed on TV and the TV station brought in the top cancer expert in Australia to challenge them. His name, Professor Boyer. Boyer disagreed with the study and said it should not have included persons not qualifying for chemotherapy, stating the actual number was 6 percent!

If you still are not convinced, see also Scientific American magazine, 1985, Volume 253, No. 5, where John Cairns writes that chemotherapy is only effective in 2 to 3 percent of cases. There are many more studies.

The fact remains. If the cause of cancer were truly addressed in a treatment or corrective action, then 5-year survivability should be 90 percent or higher.

The most common cancer treatment in current medical practice is chemotherapy. Chemotherapy basically is administering highly toxic substances to the cancer cells, which kills them. The theory is: When the cancer cells die, new healthy cells will grow in their place. It is now known that these toxic chemotherapy compounds used to treat cancer actually function by increasing the amount of superoxide in all cells! The cancer cells have less protection against superoxide and die. There is only one problem. If a patient's diet is lacking in necessary compounds like copper and manganese, the patients remaining healthy cells are vulnerable to the superoxide produced by chemotherapy and also can become cancerous.

Some of the issues with chemotherapy include:

The treatment is extremely severe and has extreme and painful side effects such as migraine headaches, hair loss, constant vomiting, vision and hearing problems and can lead to disfiguring surgeries such as mastectomies and prostatectomies.

Chemotherapy pumps unnatural, unhealthy toxins into your body promoting superoxide growth that also attacks previously healthy cells.

Chemotherapy prevents the bone marrow from making white blood cells so your immune system is lowered, increasing your risk of life-threatening infections such as pneumonia, tuberculosis or hepatitis.

The American diet is depleted of copper and manganese because of industrialized agriculture. Chemotherapy is used to destroy abnormal cells caused by insufficient nutrition.

The natural and normal way to prevent and treat cancer is to give the cells what they need to function normally and not increase already high levels of superoxide to even more dangerous levels.

Regrettably, any treatment of cancer with anything else but chemotherapy is considered unethical by the present medical establishment and government. Therefore, there are no reports in the literature of people being treated and cured of cancer by correcting their intake of copper or even manganese — except one case by Dr. Fukumi Morishige[26] who had been following research done on copper. His report in the Journal of Nutrition, Growth and Cancer, 1983, can be found at the UCLA Southern Regional Library Facility, as well as in many other medical libraries.

A 34-year-old mother of two children was admitted to Dr. Morishige's hospital at Fukuoka University (only 90 miles [a two-hour drive] from Nagasaki by the way) in October of 1981 with intolerable pain in her left upper arm (painkillers did not help). After the appropriate tests specific for cancer, she was found to have bone cancer in her upper arm.

The survivability of bone cancer is found to be poor, and standard treatment is chemotherapy and painful and radical surgery on the bone tumor. In the past, amputation had been used as a treatment for bone cancer. On November 27 of that same year, Dr. Morishige started the patient on 20 milligrams of copper sulfate, which contains about five milligrams per day of copper. This amount is easily obtained from food if you know the right foods to eat. In this case, five ounces of liver, oysters or sesame seeds would be the equivalent. He also prescribed 10 grams of vitamin C by intravenous. (We will discuss vitamin C in the following chapters and explain how it both strengthens the bones and empowers the immune system.)

Note

Copper sulfate is a chemical form of copper and not the way the body naturally gets its copper, but it was effective for this woman.

This amount is not huge; Dr. Schep took 2.5 grams of vitamin C for several years at age 60 to strengthen his bones for football.

By the end of December, 1981, the patient's pain had decreased. Up until this time, Dr. Morishige had given his patient nothing more than what you can get from your kitchen and a bottle of vitamin C pills. The woman's bone had not started to heal yet, but would given enough time. (It took Dr. Schep several years on copper and vitamin C to get his bones young again.)

To speed the healing of the patient's bone, injections of a copper amino acid complex, similar to the form of copper found in the body, were administered into an artery under the arm twice a week.

The November photo shows a tumor destroying almost a third of her upper arm. On April 29 the following year, the woman was discharged from the hospital. The April 29 photo shows a perfect, strong upper arm with no sign of disease.

The woman continued to take 20 milligrams of copper sulfate and six grams of vitamin C a day and, almost two years later at her last check-up, she was completely healthy.

In Chapter Three, we will show you how to get this same amount of copper naturally from your food.

CURING CANCER

In the present medical atmosphere, Americans are faced with considerable obstacles when trying to participate in their own treatment plans and seeking alternative treatment methods. Dr. Schep is in regular contact with anti-aging medical doctors who are using alternative cancer therapies, and they are constantly being attacked by their peers and the medical field in general.

For example, if a physician parent has a child with cancer and refuses immediate chemotherapy in lieu of seeking other, natural alternatives, that parent is in danger of being arrested for negligence and child abuse. At that time, the child would be placed in state custody and forced to begin chemotherapy treatments. As discussed earlier, chemotherapy can kill a cell that is weakened by copper deficiency. Chemotherapy also harms normal cells. Our recommendations? If you are still convinced that conventional chemotherapy is your only hope, at the minimum, immediately begin to supplement your body with copper by taking foods or the copper amino acid chelate, which contains at least five milligrams of copper (preferably 10 milligrams) and vitamin C.

The increase in copper will boost the amount of superoxide dismutase in the cells and make you less susceptible to the toxic effects of chemotherapy. If appropriate for your situation, resist surgery by showing that tumor growth has stopped or the tumor is decreasing in size.

Most likely, if you go to your doctor and ask him if increasing your daily intake of copper and vitamin C would help fight the cancer, your doctor probably will tell you that it is not necessary. Unfortunately, physicians are not trained or encouraged to research the subject of copper nutrition and cancer cells. If you show your doctor the references in this book, they may not immediately be able to understand the information, but hopefully with your encouragement, they will be motivated to try the alternative treatment before moving on to more aggressive, chemically laden options.

The bottom line: Instead of destroying cells that have become cancerous because they have too little copper in them through chemotherapy, we should bring cells back to normal by restoring their copper nutrition to adequate levels, thereby allowing the cells to function normally again.

The other major cancer treatment is surgery. This also is ridiculous. You are cutting out cancer cells because they lack copper. This will not stop the cancer — the cells in the rest of the body eventually will become cancerous, too, if copper deficiency is not addressed. The surgeon's argument: If we don't cut out the tumor, it will metastasize (spread cancer cells to the rest of the body). This is not true. If you are copper deficient, all the cells in your body can become cancerous, and removing the ones that are already cancerous will not change this.

PREVENT CANCER, JUST BY EATING!

We do not prescribe, treat or recommend in this book. All we do is point out the scientific evidence — chemotherapy and surgery will not make any difference. It ultimately is your choice. We point out that the true effect is to change your diet and include copper, manganese, selenium and anti-oxidants. This will lower free-radical damage to your cells. We prefer copper, manganese and selenium to anti-oxidants because anti-oxidants are gone within hours of eating, where hard minerals are not. But anti-oxidants are of benefit, too. What have you got to lose?

The prevention of cancer is much easier than you might think. In the following nutrition section, we will list the foods that don't contain copper. The worst offenders are white sugar, white rice, white flour, corn-fed beef and pork, produce grown by industrialized agriculture and most processed foods.

Prevention starts by simply making small changes to your diet to ensure you are getting the proper amount of daily nutrition (preferably around three to five milligrams of copper a day), which can easily be done by incorporating liberal amounts of sesame products, blackstrap molasses and nuts. We hope you acquire a taste for other great foods high in copper, including the occasional piece of shellfish (oysters are a great source of copper) and liver. Prepared correctly, oysters and liver can taste just as good as they are for your body — We promise!

It has been shown that people ingesting large quantities of grilled, fried, and/or barbecued meats have a higher tendency to develop cancer. The intense heat used in these cooking methods causes the protein in the meat to form cancerous compounds called "polycyclic aromatic hydrocarbons." Polycyclic aromatic hydrocarbons cause more superoxide to form in the body. (E. D. Werts[27]).

Likewise, people whose diets lack cruciferous vegetables tend to be more susceptible to cancer; these vegetables have very powerful anti-cancer substances in them. Cruciferous vegetables contain more phytochemicals than other groups of vegetables and they include: cabbage, bok choy, collards, broccoli, cauliflower, kale, mustard greens, arugula and kohlrabi. One of the best things you can do for yourself and your family, is also one of the most delicious. Make a delicious steak, medium or, even better, medi-

um rare, with a side of al dente broccoli and cauliflower, maybe some kale, and voila! A cancer-fighting, delicious, and easy to prepare meal.

Homemade usually is better. Make homemade coleslaw and reap the benefits of raw foods, make sauerkraut or kimchee and increase your intake of anti-cancer substances. Instructions for making homemade sauerkraut are in Chapter 10. It's really easy! It's the Chop, Salt, Stomp and Seal (CSSS) method.

We also have found that individuals with low carotene (carotene is the vegetable form of vitamin A) intake are more susceptible to cancer, as are people consuming high levels of white sugar.

Selenium, another important dietary supplement, has been shown to reduce superoxides and fight cancer. Selenium is part of an enzyme in the body called glutathione peroxidase. Its function is to destroy lipid peroxides, a chemical name for rancid fat. The outer membranes of cells are made of lipids (fats), and the enzyme protects the cell membrane. Selenium also converts hydrogen peroxide to water. The recommended daily allowance is 200 micrograms, but most American only ingest roughly 60 to 100 micrograms in their daily diet.

If peroxides are not destroyed, they can form superoxide and increase the levels of superoxide in the cells, and in our discussion on copper, we have shown that cells with high superoxide levels are cancerous. This works almost like a snowball effect, as the primary cause of high superoxide in cells is a lack of superoxide dismutase, which is caused by a lack of copper. In light of that, we highly recommend consuming foods high in selemium as an additional insurance policy against cancer.

Adequate amount s of selenium are required for an effective thyroid gland.

BENEFITS OF SELENIUM

A paper written by L.C. Clark in 1996 found that 300 micrograms of selenium was the most beneficial amount to reduce cancer. In 200 animal studies, approximately 67 percent found that selenium intake reduced the development of tumors.

We recommend a "cancer prevention diet" that includes adequate daily levels of: copper, selenium, vitamin A and C, lemongrass tea and daily consumption of cruciferous vegetables (with the least amount of cooking/heating as possible). We recommend the following foods as good sources of selenium.

> Soils of the Pacific Northwest, Upper Midwest and Atlantic Coast do not contain enough selenium for growing crops that protect against selenium deficiency. In other areas, such as the Rocky Mountain States, selenium is present in elevated levels in soils and crops

The food with the highest known level of selenium is Brazil nuts. Brazil nuts contain anywhere from 200 to 500 micrograms of selenium per ounce (depending on the selenium content of the soils). A two-ounce serving of Brazil nuts is likely to supply you with all the selenium you need.

Selenium-enriched yeast is also selenium-rich. Look for yeast that has selenium in an organic form. Inorganic forms of selenium added to yeast are not recommended and especially avoided if you have wheat allergies.

Shrimp, crab, salmon and halibut are good sources of selenium, but it may take

Note

1,000 micrograms = 1 milligram, 1,000 milligrams = 1 gram, 454 grams = 1 pound.

as much as one pound of seafood to get 160 micrograms of selenium. Wild-caught shrimp, crab, salmon and halibut are best; avoid corn-fed or farm-raised, as that depletes the natural occurrence of copper and selenium. Most store-bought shrimp and salmon is farm-raised. Check your local fish market for fresher, wilder products or ask your local supermarket's meat and fish buyer to add to their selections. There also are Web sites where you can order wild varieties.

Selenium supplements also are available, our favorite being selenomethionine, a natural form of selenium.

Lemongrass is another up and coming super food. There is some discussion on the Internet that lemongrass tea is an effective cure for cancer. The claim: Lemongrass will kill cancer cells but not normal cells when they are exposed to lemongrass essential oils in cell cultures in the laboratory.

Dr. Schep examined a paper by Dudai Weinstein and others in Planta Med., 2005 (also found at many other university medical libraries). The authors found that they could kill 50 to 81 percent of leukemic cells derived from mice and humans by incubating them in a laboratory dish with lemongrass essential oil for four hours. They found that the essential oil worked by activating an enzyme inside the cell, which cuts the DNA in the cancer cell, thereby ending its life. No explanation was given as to why it did not do the same for healthy cells. It may be possible that the superoxide ion in the cancer cell reacts with the aldehyde group in the citral oil to make a peroxide (the well-known rancidity reaction) and this triggers the 3-caspase enzyme to destroy the cells, but this remains to be proved. Cancer cells have more superoxide than healthy cells because healthy cells have superoxide dismutase to neutralize the superoxide.

However, as the basic cause of cancerous cells remains superoxide dismutase deficiency due to a lack of copper, the actual correction remains — increase copper intake initially to 10 milligrams and, after cure is affected, maintain a normal healthy intake of two to four milligrams a day.

The use of lemongrass may be beneficial in accelerating the cure by destroying excess cancer cells, but the utmost concern still remains — correct copper trace mineral deficiency and thereby keep a healthy SOD level in our cells.

ALTERNATIVE THERAPIES FOR CANCER

The present day "alternative cure" literature focuses on natural cures for cancer, one being the "Macrobiotic Diet." This diet emphasizes whole grains, beans and a 30 to 40 percent vegetable intake. Whole grains instead of refined grains will almost double the copper intake, and 40 percent vegetables will load the body with anti-oxidants. This is in line with this chapter, except we emphasize even more powerful sources of copper and manganese, namely nuts, brans, oysters and liver, with beans also being a useful source of copper.

J.P. Carter[30] with the American College of Nutrition, 1993, found that the median survival rate of men with prostate cancer increased from eight years to 15 years when they went to a low-fat high-fiber reduced-calorie diet. Compare those rates to the dismal rate of chemotherapy and surgery.

Note: You will find that the use of vitamins A and C for cancer has extensive opposition in medical literature and on the Internet. We have purposefully ignored all the scientific publications attacking the usage of vitamin C, as the studies ignore positive results and these papers are promoted by the pharmaceutical companies that oppose normal natural healing methods. Dr. Schep communicated with Dr. Linus Pauling (personal correspondence) on the superiority of copper over vitamin C as it is a more persistent superoxide scavenger in the body than C and he has remained a proponent of vitamin C during his lifetime.

ARTHRITIS

We are getting arthritis from a *lack of* omega-3 fatty acids and *too much* omega-6 fatty acids in our diets. And we're here to show you that inflammation in the body causes arthritis, painkillers promote arthritis, and omega-3 fatty acids are the true natural anti-inflammatories for your body. (Omega-6 fatty acids promote inflammation.)

> "I was born to run free
> Across the prairie
> With the grass
> Waving at my knee
> And the buffalo will come again
> Down from the sky
> To run with me"
> — (R.A.S)

The remedy we promote involves: discontinuing painkillers; increasing intake of omega-3 oil to lessen inflammation of the joints; taking chondroitin and glucosamine to heal cartilage; exercising to stimulate formation of cartilage; taking MSM (a form of sulfur) to strengthen ligaments, and vitamin C to promote the formation of collagen.

It is estimated that 35 million Americans suffer from arthritis. Medical science's only answer is to take non-steroidal anti-inflammatory drugs (NSAIDS), a form of painkillers, which only make you more and more dependent on them. You will be stunned to learn that as many as five studies have proven NSAIDS actually worsen your joint damage, eventually leading to joint replacement surgery.

If you or someone you know is suffering from arthritis, you know that running free through a grassy field, buffalo or not, can be slow, painful and maybe even impossible.

Most forms of arthritis are considered to be caused by inflammation, and, at present, are being treated by synthetic drug suppression and joint replacement surgery, neither of which is natural or satisfactory.

It is easy to lose hope when you are in pain and the treatments prescribed fail to lessen the pain and decreased mobility. Facing surgery can be a scary and expensive option and sometimes seems like the only way, especially since arthritis can be completely debilitating. However, what if you could eliminate inflammation and increase mobility safely, effectively and without the expense and risk of surgery? YOU CAN! Dr. Schep is a prime example of someone who suffered from intense arthritis pain and he is here to show you how you, too, can take back your life. Seven years ago he started playing rugby at the age of 56. By some unconscious innate plan that activity landed him in an orthopedic specialists office and, coincidentally, spurred the writing of this book.

The Center for Disease Control (CDC) reports that 46 million people in the United States have been told they have arthritis. That's a ratio of 1-to-6! The CDC also reports that Americans spend $81 billion per year on treatment for arthritis. The loss of earnings due to the symptoms of arthritis is $108 billion per year.

Within three months of beginning to play rugby, Dr. Schep found himself in the specialists office with two severely swollen knees. After having an MRI, he was told that he had arthritis and would never be able to run again, let alone play rugby. The specialist indicated that cycling and swimming were the only exercises that were safe for his condition. He also told Dr. Schep that he was a prime candidate for knee replacement surgery because the cartilage in his knees had worn away. He was told to return to the specialist's office in six weeks for a checkup.

At the six-week checkup, Dr. Schep shocked the specialist and prompted him to make the comment "Wow, come up with a cure and we could make millions!" The cure we now have (keep reading for the secret). And the millions? Well, maybe someday.

DR. SCHEP IS A HUMAN STUDY

As a teacher of nutrition and a doctorate chemist, Dr. Schep started to search for the cause and cure for arthritis the same day the doctor diagnosed him with arthritis. What he researched and found: You can substantially improve joint health and manage it to a point where you can live a normal, healthy, comfortable life and — even participate in championship sports. The only way to do this is through natural supplements, and that requires the absolute avoidance of drugs and surgery. Dr. Schep, of course, tested his research on himself and he gives us the following testimonial:

"Three months after my arthritis diagnosis, I showed up for rugby practice with new knee cartilage in both knees and I have not missed a Division I or Division II rugby game in seven years.

I play for a U.S. Division I team, and I am a member of the top Super League team in the United States of America, Belmont Shore Rugby Club." (The Rugby Super League is organized and sanctioned by USA Rugby as the premier level of men's club competition in the USA).

I train (and play) shoulder to shoulder with players representing the USA internationally. This afternoon, before settling in to work on this book, I played as captain of a team that included four international players — players that have played in front of tens of thousands — all the way from Hong Kong to Dubai.

It is unheard of for a 63-year-old to be playing championship rugby. It normally is not possible for someone my age to play rugby at this high level with teammates three times younger than myself, nor has it been done before.

A 63-year-old person with a 'normal' American diet and exercise routine would suffer from severe injuries, broken bones, joint damage (also known as arthritis), not to mention cardiovascular problems and shortness of breath, angina, torn and swollen ligaments and muscular weakness if rough-housing around and participating in brutal tackles with full-grown 20 to 30-year-old men. I actually had complaints from the coach, Matt Webber, that I was too rough on the players during training, and these are tough, world-class, young professional athletes! Must be rough getting beat up by a

63-year-old, but somebody has to do it!

Not only that, I also kick for the team. There probably is no more stress and shock to the knees than kicking a rugby ball, heavier than an American football, over the poles from 30 yards away. I tend to kick with the toe instead of the side of the foot, even more shock."

All the books available today on arthritis have been written by armchair specialists, in other words, people who just speculate and brainstorm about the causes and cures of arthritis, but don't actively participate in finding and trying cures. The arthritis cure you are about to read has been born, raised and put to the test in the most extreme ways possible, namely championship football and extreme fitness training, requiring running flat out for hours on end by a subject over 60 years old.

We are going to teach you, too, how to have your knees and hips escape the knife of the surgeon and lead a pain-free and physically active life. You may not want to play football, but you most certainly may want to garden, go walking, jogging or running, go on long hikes, play social tennis and lead an active life. And this system works. Dr. Schep knows — he did it! The reason it works: It removes the actual, true cause of arthritis, not just the symptoms. Want the cure? Keep reading!

TOSS THE PAIN RELIEVERS
If you have arthritis, or if you are experiencing joint problems or pain at any age (we have seen school children wearing knee and ankle supports while participating in activities like soccer, track, basketball, etc.), the first thing you should do is toss that bot-

tle of painkillers in the garbage. We know, it feels like your salvation at this point, but trust us. Take a look in your medicine cabinet or kitchen cupboard and throw away any over-the-counter or doctor prescribed painkillers. Gather up all of them and toss them right out. Non-steroidal anti-inflammatory drugs, or NSAIDS, are currently the prescribed, official treatment for arthritis, but they are unnatural, unhealthy and very hard on your body.

Some of the reasons we ask you to throw them away include:

NSAIDS injure (eat away) at your stomach lining.

NSAIDS increase inflammation in the body, even in arteries, which elevates your cardiovascular risk.

NSAIDS aggravate your joints, which makes the pain and inflammation even greater, causing you to take even higher doses to alleviate the pain and stiffness. (Great for pharmaceutical company profits, but bad for your overall health and well being.)

NSAIDS are made of synthetic materials and as such are not beneficial to your body in any way.

It is sad that today the role of the healer, which is to promote the normal healing process, does not occur in the drug and medical treatment of arthritis. Current arthritis treatments do not remove the cause of the disease, nor do they assist the body with the natural healing process once the cause of the disease is removed. Sadly, drug treatments not only *do not* promote the body's powerful healing process, they actually work against the body's natural process and negate any positive improvement by adding detrimental chemicals to the mix.

While NSAIDS or painkillers may provide you with temporary respite from pain and swelling, they are just masking the symptoms of the disease. The painkillers work by blocking prostaglandins, which are hormone-like substances that contribute to pain, inflammation, fever and muscle cramps. In order to do this, they are designed to interfere with the natural process of omega fatty acid metabolism in the body. The omega-6 oils in our diet *increase* inflammatory substances; the omega-3 oils *decrease* inflammatory substances.

"Prostaglandins" in our body are made from omega-3, unfortunately, NSAIDS interfere with both inflammatory and anti-inflammatory substances in the body.

Some of these hormones called "cytokines" prevent inflammation of the joints, others prevent inflammation of the stomach, the liver, and some prevent inflammation of the arteries and veins.

In some circumstances cytokines increase inflammation in the stomach, kidneys or liver. Pro- or anti-inflammatory cytokines are produced by the immune system, as opposed to regular hormones that are produced by the glands.

Once the painkillers or anti-inflammatory medications wear off (or when you stop taking them) the pain, stiffness and swelling come right back with a vengeance. It also means that while temporarily relieving pain and swelling, you could be causing damage to other parts of your body. Unfortunately, the more effective (stronger) the NSAIDS, the greater the risk of causing serious damage to your stomach, liver, kidneys and joints. Sadly, the better the NSAID works the greater its strength, which means greater and longer-lasting damage to your internal organs.

NSAIDS also can cause some very serious allergic reactions, including, but not limited to, rashes, swelling of the face and neck, difficulty breathing and shock. Currently, the Federal Drug Administration (FDA) has asked pharmaceutical companies to include a warning on their NSAID medication pamphlets and packaging stating that consuming NSAIDS can increase the risk of cardiovascular events and potentially life-threatening gastrointestinal bleeding. The FDA is also asking manufacturers of all over-the-counter NSAIDS (i.e. Aleve®, Advil®) to revise labels to include more specific information about potential cardiovascular and gastrointestinal risks as well as the risk of potential skin reactions.

As one drug company just found out, NSAIDS absolutely cannot be used by people with cardiovascular problems. This particular company recently had a billion dollar court judgment entered against them for their brand-specific NSAID painkiller causing the death of a patient due to cardiovascular complications.

The side effects of NSAIDS can be extremely severe, but doctors are still prescribing them at an alarming rate. The consensus in the medical community is that if the patient is made fully aware of the risks, it is acceptable to continue writing prescriptions for NSAIDS. This is a dangerous situation. Most patients rely on their doctors to help guide them to medications that will cure, heal or greatly improve their ailments and conditions.

We believe that our medical community has a personal interest in each of us as a patient and that they would never prescribe medications that could prove to be harmful. So while we hear a list of side effects,

we don't believe they are as serious as they sound, since our trusted doctor is recommending we take them. Due to the risks associated with their use, some professionals will not prescribe oral NSAIDS, but continue to use them via injection, creams, lotions and topical gels. While this does reduce the risks, it will not prevent the damage caused to the joints, liver and stomach — it is still absorbed into the body.

The drug companies of course are fully aware of the damaging effects of their NSAIDS. So, they tried to rectify the situation by making pain relievers that do not inhibit the Cox-1 enzymes, which lessen inflammation in the body as opposed to Cox-2 enzymes, which promote inflammation. COX stands for cyclo-oxgenase and is the name of the enzyme that makes prostaglandins from omega-3 and omega-6 acids. More on this later.

Cox-1 enzymes protect the stomach and work by inhibiting the Cox-2 enzymes that cause inflammation. Cox-2 enzyme inhibitors reduce inflammation by blocking the final step in the arachidonic acid series to form the Series 2 prostaglandins, which are inflammatory. Unfortunately, while the Cox-2 enzymes block the production of inflammatory prostaglandins, they also block the production of the anti-inflammatory Series-3 prostaglandins that are made from omega-3 fatty acids that we get from the oils and fats in our diet. Correcting the balance of omega-3 and omega-6 fatty acids in the diet solves the inflammation problem naturally and avoids all the pitfalls of the NSAIDS.

While it is easy to read this information, it can be hard to put into practical use when at the doctor's office, pharmacy, or staring

Traditional NSAIDS

CHEMICAL NAME	TRADE NAME(S)
Diclofenac	Voltaren, Cataflam
Diflunisal	Dolobid
Etodolac	Lodine
Flurbiprofen	Ansaid
Ibuprofen	Motrin, Advil
Indomethacin	Indocin
Ketoprofen	Orudis, Oruvail
Ketorolac	Toradol
Nabumetone	Relafen
Naproxen	Naprosyn, Aleve
Oxaprozin	Daypro
Piroxicam	Feldene
Sulindac	Clinoril
Tolmetin	Tolectin

Cox-2 Inhibitors

Celecoxib	Celebrex
Refocoxib	Vioxx (this has been withdrawn from the market)

ACETYLSALICYLATES AND SALICYLATES

Aspirin	Motrin, Bayer, Ecotrin, St. Joseph
Methly Salicylate	Bengay
Magnesium Salicylate	Doans
Acetaminophen	Tylenol, Excedrin
Trolamine Salicylate	Aspercreme

The following are not NSAIDS, nor a replacement for omega-3 fatty acids

Menthol	Bengay, Tiger Balm
(E)-N-(4-Hydroxy-3-methoxybenzyl	Capsaicin

down the pain-reliever aisle at the grocery store. To take out the guesswork, we have included the easy-to-follow table at left, which outlines the type of pain reliever, the drug name and the common shelf/pharmacy names.

In summary, the disadvantages of NSAIDS:

Stomach disorders.

Kidney disorders.

Induces/contributes to high blood pressure.

Accelerates joint degeneration.

Causes ulceration and bleeding of the stomach lining.

Causes "leaky gut syndrome," which occurs when the NSAID creates tiny, pinpoint perforations in the surface of the small intestine.

Weakens the intestinal barrier.

INCORPORATE OMEGA-3 FATTY ACIDS

To start increasing your body's ability to heal and relieve pain on its own, you must immediately up your daily intake of omega-3 fatty acids to your diet. You will need approximately 5,000 milligrams per day.

What Are Omega-3 and Omega-6 Fatty Acids?

Omega-3 and omega-6 fatty acids come from the oils and fats in our diet. Omega-3 fatty acids consist of alpha linolenic acid called "ALA," eicosapentaenoic acid called "EPA," docosapentaenoic acid called "DPA," and docosahexaenoic acid called "DHA."

We get these from two sources — animals or vegetables. Vegetable oils contain only ALA, which must be converted by the body into EPA, DPA and DHA, the forms

the body needs to *suppress inflammation.*

EPA, DPA, and DHA are contained in animal fats. Their big advantage is that *the body can use them directly* without having to make them from ALA.

Omega-6 fatty acid consists of linoleic acid or "LA." Note carefully that the name differs from ALA (alpha *linolenic* acid). There is no "n" after the "e."

LA also occurs in vegetable oils. LA and ALA both are known as essential fatty acids, because the body cannot make these and must get them from the diet. Safflower (high oleic) and olive oil are extremely rich in oleic acid also called omega-9 fatty acid. It is less widely known that *omega-9 fatty acid is also an inflammation fighter and similar to omega-3 fatty acids.*

Why Do We Need Omega-3 Acids?

Omega-3 fatty acids help relieve arthritis pain by lessening the amount of inflammation and swelling in our bodies, while omega-6 fatty acids increase the amount of inflammation in our bodies. *Our modern diets have become so unbalanced* that we are ingesting high amounts of omega-6, and not nearly enough omega-3. This is the main reason why so many people are suffering from arthritis, and why they are starting to suffer at much younger ages than previous generations.

To overcome this, we must increase the good omega-3 fatty acids and decrease the amount of omega-6 fatty acids in our diet. As we discussed earlier, omega-3 fatty acids are the natural replacements for harmful painkillers and anti-inflammatory drugs (NSAIDS) that we use to suppress inflammation, but that have harmful effects on the body, including actually worsening the joints.

Incorporating omega-3 into your diet is extremely important as it will radically improve the body's health and manage inflammation in the body. Once this is achieved, other healthy supplements will further build on and improve health and joint strength. Arthritis is inflammation that has become out of control and it must be stopped. Inflammation can and does have its function in the body for limited purposes, but it must not proceed unchecked and out of control.

When you ingest omega-3 fatty acids, they are converted by enzymes in the body into anti-inflammatory hormones called prostaglandins and leukotrienes, which decrease inflammation in the body and joints, as well as protect the lining of the stomach. As a side benefit, they also *decrease inflammation in the veins and arteries*, which helps the cardiovascular system.

On the other hand, ingested omega-6 fatty acids convert to arachidonic acids, which promote inflammation in the body. The majority of omega-6 fatty acids we consume come from vegetable oils, lard and egg yolks. The linoleic (LA) acid in the oils is converted to gamma-linolenic acid (GLA) in the body and is then broken down into arachidonic acid (AA). Excess amounts of LA and AA are unhealthy because they *promote inflammation.*

This means diets that include more omega-6 oils than omega-3 oils stimulate the pro-inflammatory processes in the body, while diets that include more omega-3s stimulate anti-inflammatory processes. It is important to mention that both omega-3 and omega-6 oils are essential for human health, but finding the appropriate balance of the two is extremely important.

Too much omega-6 in the body can create a situation that promotes chronic inflammation, propagation of cancer, heart disease, stroke, diabetes and arthritis. The body's anti-inflammatory responses are intimately regulated by omega-3s. The purpose of inflammation is to deal with acute injury or a microbial attack. However, inflammation must not be allowed to proceed to excess levels or to become uncontrolled. If the inflammatory response is needlessly provoked, damage to tissue, joints and organs of the body occur. The shortage of omega-3 fatty acids in the diet of the industrialized nations (North America is a great example), has created a situation of chronic inflammation. Normal, then unchecked inflammation levels precede and lead to arthritis, which leads to a vicious, never-ending circle of inflammation and disease treated by harmful chemicals that cause more inflammation and have serious health risks.

The following is under authority from the Canadian Asthma Prevention Institute. Why the Canadian Asthma Prevention Institute? Because inflammation due to lack

Function of an Enzyme

The function of an enzyme in the body is to make it easier for the body to perform chemical reactions to make substances required for the body. In the case where the body makes anti-inflammatory hormones, it uses a COX enzyme. COX stands for cyclo-oxgenase and is the name of the enzyme that makes prostaglandins from omega-3 and omega-6 acids. There are many enzymes in the body, for example, the collagenase enzyme, which destroys aged collagen in the body. Too much of this can also cause inflammation and arthritis.

of omega-3 is not restricted to joints. It also can appear in the lungs and the bronchi, depending in the individual.

WHAT HAPPENS TO OMEGA-3 FATTY ACIDS IN THE BODY?

When alpha linolenic acid (ALA) is ingested, it is converted to EPA in the body by enzymes. (These enzymes require sufficient amounts of vitamin C, B6, niacin [B3], magnesium and zinc.) One enzyme that helps with this conversion is *delta-5-saturase.* A very important enzyme that is either friend or foe.

This same enzyme (*delta-5-saturase)* converts the EPA into type-3 prostaglandins, which reduce inflammation. Deficiencies in the above vitamins and minerals can interfere with this conversion. Also important is the COX-1 enzyme in the body. COX-1 enzyme also helps convert the EPA into Series 3 anti-inflammatory prostaglandins.

Our bodies have both COX-1 and COX-2 enzymes and prescription drugs or NSAIDS, such as ibuprofen, aspirin, naproxen and diclofenac inhibit the COX-1 enzyme. The NSAIDS interfere with the natural anti-inflammatory process by suppressing the COX-1 enzyme, which also protects our stomach lining. Ingesting omega-3 results in the reduction of inflammation.

Simply stated, painkillers suppress inflammation in the body. They suppress the COX-2 enzyme and inhibit the natural anti-inflammatory process by suppressing the COX-1 enzyme. This results in exposing the stomach lining and the liver to inflammation and the joints to continued inflammation and deterioration. Omega-3 naturally suppresses inflammation in the body but it does not destroy the stomach lining, harm the liver or destroy the joints.

The omega-6 fatty acid, linoleic acid, (LA) is converted by the enzymes in the body into two things. The first is Series-1 prostaglandins; these are anti-inflammatory. The second is the conversion of LA into arachidonic acid (AA). Our friendly omega-3 enzyme, *delta-5-saturase*, does this conversion.

Arachidonic acid (AA) also is converted to Series-2 prostaglandins by the COX -2 enzyme. These are inflammatory! The COX-2 enzyme is inhibited by NSAIDS. This is why NSAIDS work — inhibiting inflammation; but inhibiting the COX-1 enzyme also does additional damage to the body.

When not enough omega-3 fatty acids are ingested, the delta-5 saturase enzyme is no longer able to convert ALA into EPA. Therefore, more omega-6 (LA) is converted by the delta-5 saturase enzyme into arachidonic acid (AA), which in turn goes to the inflammatory Series-2 prostaglandins.

This means a lack of omega-3 fatty acids in the diet results in a double whammy. *Less* of the Series-3 anti-inflammatory prostaglandins are produced from the omega-3 fatty acids and *more* inflammatory Series-2 prostaglandins are produced from the omega 6 fatty acids.

Notes

This trial indicated there was a 36 percent conversion of LA to EPA from flaxseed oil in the body.

The international panel of essential fatty acid experts in the Journal of the American College of Nutrition recommend a 1-1 ratio of omega-6 to omega-3.

STUDIES OF OMEGA-3 SUPPLEMENTATION

G. E. Caughey[31] and other doctors/scientists in the American Journal of Clinical Nutrition 1996, p116-122, state that fish oil, or in the absence thereof, flaxseed oil, can be very effective in anti-inflammatory (and anti-atherosclerotic) diets.

In their study, they gave a group of people 14 grams of flaxseed oil per day. This supplied the body with good levels of ALA, which is converted by the body to EPA, the body-beneficial omega-3 fatty acid.

They gave another group sunflower oil, which essentially only supplies omega-6 fatty acid (LA). After only four weeks, they found that the flaxseed group had 30 percent less inflammation-promoting compounds in the body than the sunflower group.

Then, they switched both the flaxseed oil and the sunflower oil groups to 9 grams of fish oil per day for four weeks and found a 70 to 80 percent reduction of inflammation-promoting compounds in the body.

THE OMEGA-6 AND OMEGA-3 RATIO IN THE DIET

The average daily intake of the omega-3 oils EPA and DHA combined is approximately 130 milligrams in North America. Various authorities recommend anything from a ratio of 1-to-1 to a ratio of 3-to-1.

That's 520 milligrams short of published recommendations, and 870 milligrams short of the 1,000 milligrams recommended by the American Heart Association in cases of heart disease!

As our goal is to put a stop to the inflammation associated with arthritis, we recommend (at least until inflammation is halted) that you maintain at least a 1-1 ratio.

To help you increase your intake of omega-3 fatty acids, we list the following sources:

Fish oil

Salmon oil

Krill oil

Flaxseed oil

Wild Fish

Eggs, special omega-3 enriched

Mayonnaise (safflower or canola) and olive oil. (Safflower and olive are rich in omega-9, which has the same benefit as omega-3 fatty acids.)

Decreasing your omega-6 intake may include reducing the following foods:

Cereals

Whole-grain breads

Baked goods

Fried food

Margarine

Most vegetable oils: grape seed, canola, sunflower, coconut, etc.

Corn-fed beef

Corn-fed farm-raised fish

With the exception of fresh seaweed, plants rarely contain EPA or DHA. The best source of omega-3, by far, is wild salmon. Cold-water fish, fresh seaweed, tuna, krill and mackerel also are good sources of omega-3. Farmed salmon tend to be inactive and overfed, leading their oil to be inferior to that of wild salmon. Farmed salmon also contains much higher levels of pesticides and PCBs than wild salmon.

All commercial salmon, with the exception of Alaskan salmon, are from farms. To protect their legacy of quality products, Alaskan fishermen do not allow salmon farms in Alaska.

As today's American diet consists mainly of foods containing omega-6 fatty acids and very little or no cold-water fish and fresh seaweed, our bodies tend to be subject to inflammation and arthritis due to lack of proper nutrition.

So what is the preferred way to get omega-3 oils? Fish oil or flaxseed oil? Omega-3 fatty acids are easily destroyed by heat and processing, so there are some who say it is better to get omega-3 fatty acids from flaxseed oil so that the body can make its own omega-3 acids. EPA and DHA are five times more sensitive to heat and oxygen than alpha linolenic acid, (ALA), which in turn is five times more sensitive than linoleic acid (omega-6 acid.) Fish oil is subject to rancidity and damage during processing. The truth may be that both flaxseed oil and some fish oil supplementation may be in order.

A 100-pound woman taking the recommended two tablespoons of flaxseed oil per day (one tablespoon/50 pounds of body weight per day) will provide about 14 grams (14,000 mil-

Polychlorinated Biphenyls (PCBs)

As explained: A group of manufactured chemicals including 209 different (but closely related) compounds made up of carbon, hydrogen and chlorine. If released to the environment, they persist for long periods of time and can biomagnify in the food web. They are an organic toxicant suspected of causing cancer, endocrine disruption and other adverse impacts on organisms.

— San Francisco Estuary Institute

Note

The international panel of essential fatty acid experts in the Journal of the American College of Nutrition recommend a 1-1 ratio of omega-6 to omega-3.

Fish Oil vs. Flaxseed

ADVANTAGES OF FISH OIL
Provides EPA and DHA directly to the body without need for conversion.
Assimilated easier by men.

DISADVANTAGES OF FISH OIL
Tends to be contaminated with polychlorinated biphenyls (PCBs), mercury, organochlorine pesticides and dioxin. Can be degraded during the processing needed to remove these pollutants.
They have much greater susceptibility to rancidity than flaxseed's alpha linolenic acid, so may be less potent than claimed.
Assimilated less by women.

ADVANTAGES OF FLAXSEED OIL
Less subject to rancidity than fish oil, allowing a much better chance for potency. Can be kept free of pesticides and pollutants if grown completely organically.
Assimilated easier by women.

DISADVANTAGES OF FLAXSEED OIL
Must be converted by the body to omega-3 fatty acids (with the help of proper nutrition). Good vitamin and mineral nutrition required to affect conversion.
Assimilated less easily by men.

ligrams) of alpha linolenic acid (ALA).

At the 36 percent conversion rate, 14,000 milligrams of alpha linolenic acid produces a total of 5,000 milligrams of omega-3; 2,940 milligrams of EPA; 840 milligrams of DPA; and 1,260 milligrams of DHA. This is the equivalent of about 17 large 1,000-milligram capsules of fish oil (each containing 300 milligrams of EPA and DHA, which is close to twice as much as the highest recommended therapeutic dose of fish oil.

KRILL OIL

Krill oil is an amazing food, courtesy of the ocean. Krill oil has 0.8 percent alpha linolenic acid (ALA); 14.7 percent eicosapentaenoic acid (EPA); 14.7 percent DPA; 8.3 percent docosahexaenoic acid (DHA); and it contains 100 parts per million (ppm) of astaxanthin, an orange-colored material that is a powerful protectant and anti-oxidant. The advantage of this compound — together with other anti-oxidants — it protects and stabilizes the omega-3 acids, which are very unstable. This orange and pink-colored astaxanthin causes the pink color in salmon. The oil is one-third omega-3, one-third phosphatidyl choline, and one-third phospholipids. The ratio of omega-6 to omega-3 is only parts to 100 parts. It is similar or as superior, as fish oil for a source of omega-3. However, it is superior to fish oil with its protective anti-oxidants and phospholipids, which help the body better utilize the omega-3 acids.

Sometimes, adding new supplements to your diet can be very costly, but omega-3 supplements tend to cost very little. A few cents per day for strong, healthy, pain-free joints is a small price to pay! We went to some major big-box stores to research the

The Oxygen Radical Absorbance Capability (ORAC)

This is a measurement of the anti-oxidant power of a substance. The higher the number — the more resistant the substance is to rancidity. The relative values for oils are as follows:
Fish oil: 8
Coenzyme Q10: 11
Astaxanthin: 51
Lycophene: 58
Krill oil: 378
The table shows that omega-3 fatty acids in krill oil are more protected against rancidity by anti-oxidants, and secondly, that krill oil also supplies powerful anti-oxidants to the body to protect the cells and the fatty acids in the body.

cost of oils and found the following prices to be good cost averages:

Fish oil capsules: 250 soft-gel capsules averaged approximately $0.45 per day (10 soft gels per day).

Flaxseed oil capsules: 300 soft-gel capsules averaged approximately $0.86 per day (13 capsules per day).

Flaxseed oil: Approximately $0.72 per ounce (one ounce per day).

Seal oil (Canada only): 24 capsules at 500 milligrams each averaged approximately $1.99 per day (one capsule per day). *Note: Seal oil is banned by anti-hunting groups in the U.S.*

Krill oil: 60 soft gel capsules at 500 milligrams each averaged $6.66 per day (20 soft gels per day).

OUR RECOMMENDED SUPPLEMENTS
No. 1: Krill oil.

Krill oil is extremely expensive in comparison to other supplements. To get the recommended 10,000 milligrams of krill oil per day, you would need to take 20 capsules, 500 milligrams each, which would cost roughly $200 per month. Compared to the $15,000 to $30,000 cost of knee or hip replacement surgery (not to mention the pain, rehabilitation, time off, etc.), it is a small expense. However, in these tough economic times, $200 per month can make a serious dent in your monthly budget.

No. 2: Fish and krill oil combined.

A great, cost-efficient alternative is to take seven 1,000-milligram capsules of fish oil concentrate per day (approx. $0.25) along with two 500-milligram capsules of krill oil (approx. $0.67). For under a dollar a day, you will benefit from the powerful anti-oxidants and emulsifiers found in the krill oil and also benefit from the properties of the fish oil.

Once your joints have healed, you can reduce your daily intake of omega-3 fatty acids to approximately 2,500 milligrams. You should keep taking this supplement for as long as you want healthy joints (forever, right?). Any continuance of NSAIDS will severely reduce the effectiveness of this cure.

Here are some of the main reasons this cure works:

1. Omega-3 oil releases anti-inflammatory agents in your body.

2. Inflammation in your body and your joints originally was caused by a *lack of omega-3 fatty acids* in your diet, NOT by a lack of artificial NSAIDS.

3. There are no, or very little, omega-3 fatty acids in the American diet.

4. Omega-3 oil will stop inflammation in your joints and cause them to become normal again, like the good-old-days when you were a kid and your joints could take a lot of pounding.

The bottom line: Deal with arthritis the correct and natural way: omega-3 oil, exercise and a healthy, vitamin- and mineral-rich diet.

RESTORATION THROUGH NUTRIENTS

The next step is to restore your joints by taking the cartilage-healing nutrients glucosamine and chondroitin sulfate until the joints are fully healed. This takes, on average, about three months. These nutrients are necessary for your body to create new cartilage. Do not, however, take these supplements while still taking NSAIDS, as the NSAIDS defeat the purpose of the supple-

Tips to Increase Your Omega-3 Intake

Purchase omega-3 eggs (sold in health food stores and high-end grocery stores. Two eggs contain about 300 milligrams of omega-3.

Use only safflower or canola mayonnaise. Canola oil has a very favorable ratio of omega-6 to omega-3 (2-to-2).

If purchasing salmon, go for wild Alaskan salmon whenever possible. Copper River salmon are our favorite. They have a long journey and travel great distances, which promotes strong, healthy muscles that contain more omega-3 oils than other salmon varieties.

Purchase grass-fed beef.

Cultivate a liking for chia seeds. They can be added to breakfast cereals. (Buckwheat, chia and chopped cashews make an excellent cereal with blackstrap molasses and milk or almond milk.)

ments. After joints are fully restored, older people should continue with the glucosamine and chondroitin sulfate supplements. As you age, cartilage can be broken down faster than your body can make it and extra glucosamine will counteract this.

STRENGTHEN YOUR LIGAMENTS

Strong ligaments are a critical part of supporting not only your joints, but your whole body. If your ligaments are weak, they cannot support your newly healed joints and you still could suffer from pain and stiffness, even risk additional injury.

The best way to strengthen your ligaments is to take an organic sulphur compound called MSM, which is the abbreviation for methyl sulfonyl methane. This is a natural nutrient that is missing from most American diets. For the first two weeks, take 1,000 milligrams per day. The third week decrease your intake to 1,000 milligrams per week.

Without the compound MSM, ligaments turn weak and are unable to support the joints by holding them in place. This contributes to joint damage, as misaligned joints are much more susceptible to wear and tear than joints that are balanced and in place. Strong, limber ligaments are especially important for those actively participating in any kind of athletics or physical activity.

Now, if your knees are severely inflamed

Note

It is not very well known that omega-9 fatty acids found in olive oil and high-oleic safflower oil (contains the highest concentration) have the same anti-inflammatory benefits as omega-3 fatty acids.

and damaged, it also may be that the joint space in your knees has become reduced. In this case, just taking MSM and omega-3 will not cure your problem.

One of the reasons joint space becomes reduced is that ligaments can shrink with age. When the ligaments shrink, they pull your leg bones together. This means that there may be no new room for cartilage to grow and there also may not be room for knee lubricating fluid, called hyaluronic acid (a slippery, mucous-like material made from glucosamine). To self-test for reduced joint space, follow these steps:

Stand next to a high-backed chair or a wall with your feet shoulder width apart.

Place one hand on the chair or wall for support and balance.

Bend the leg at the knee, opposite your support hand, towards your backside. If you cannot get your heel close to your butt and have pain, you have reduced joint space.

If possible, grasp your ankle and pull your foot towards your backside.

This test/stretch can be painful, but works to not only self-diagnose reduced joint space, but if done daily, will actually increase the joint space. Done in conjunction with the proper supplements (listed above), you can alleviate the pain, swelling and stiffness arthritis is famous for. This exercise should be done daily with each leg, gradually increasing the length of time for each stretch. Once you can just about touch your heel to your bottom, your joint space will be restored to a normal (or close to normal) amount. Then your joint should heal within six weeks. As a side note: Women or men with petite thigh muscles may need to put a small, rolled towel behind the knee to achieve the correct angle and maximum stretching. For some extra help, although painful, a holistic chiropractor will have you lie on your stomach and stretch your legs toward your bottom. However, this should not be done prior to a few weeks on MSM and omega-3. You don't want to risk further damage to weakened ligaments.

There are other, more formal ways to find out if you have reduced joint space: appointment with a holistic chiropractor, MRI or an X-Ray.

WORK IT OUT

The next step is to go jogging. Yes, you heard right — JOGGING! Not only jogging, but running, playing tennis, basketball, distance walking, playing soccer, even rugby! This may sound crazy to you, and your doctor may shake his or her head and think you have lost your mind. And he or she probably will tell you that exercise will debilitate your already sore joints. This is because the true cause and cure for arthritis has never been widely published — until now.

Arthritis and joint damage are not caused by running or walking on hard surfaces or by any form of shock from exercise or prolonged standing. Joint damage is caused by a lack of anti-inflammatory substances in the modern American diet.

Think about this: If arthritis and damaged joints were caused by exercise and shock, arthritis would be heavily present in Tarahumara Indians (Copper Canyon and Northwest Mexico), who play four-day-long soccer games that can span hundreds of miles (from Guerrero to Chihuahua). Also, wild animals like ostriches, who have very skinny, small knee joints supporting 300-pound bodies and run at high speeds for long distances to avoid being a lion's dinner, would be crippled by arthritis. Arthritis is unheard of in ostriches as well as Tarahumara Indians, at least before the Tarahumaras began adding American-grown corn oil and white sugar to their diets.

Nature, over millions of years, has designed cartilage basal cells (the cells that make cartilage) to do one thing and one thing only. The more they are pounded upon, the more cartilage tissue they make. The Stanford University paper below absolutely proved that point. Take basal cells, subject them to 1,500 pounds of pressure, and what do they do? They make three times more cartilage.

When Dr. Schep was first struck down with arthritis, his doctor at that time told him he could not run and that the best thing he could do was rest his knees. The doctor indicated that any type of running would only further damage the joints. Dr. Schep found this unacceptable and started searching for cures.

He discovered an enormously important piece of research done at Stanford University by R.L. Smith et al[32]. For the experiment, they took sample cells that manufacture cartilage (the hard, smooth, ivory-like material that protects the ends of the bones where they join together) from the joints of cattle and grew them in the lab. They fed the cells nutrients and measured the amount of cartilage they produced. Then the researchers did something surprising. They took the same cell samples, mixed in a nutrient mixture and subjected them to enormous levels of pressure — 1,500 pounds. To put that into perspective: You normally inflate your car tires to 32 pounds, so this is approximately 47 times more pressure! What did the cells do when subjected to this huge amount of pressure? They increased the rate of cartilage manufactured by a stunning 65 percent!

At first, Dr. Schep was confused. He knew if he created some sort of pressure-inducing binding device for his knee, he could easily crush it and create more permanent damage. After three days of reflection, he suddenly realized that cells, which have been making cartilage over millions of years of evolution, are designed to dramatically increase cartilage production when subjected to pressure, but the pressure needed to be internal, not external. So, how do we create internal pressure? Exercising! Running, walking, jogging, and/or jumping to be exact.

These activities subject the knees to extreme shock, banging and pressure. The knees response is to immediately start producing more cartilage. This means that the more humans and animals run and jump, the stronger the joints become. However, a caution — depriving the joints of critical omega-3, which is an anti-inflammatory, will force the body to destroy cartilage faster than the cells can make it.

Weeks after Dr. Schep had corrected his body by taking extra omega-3, glucosamine,

---

Per year, the world roughly produces:

784 million tons of corn
651 million tons of rice
607 million tons of wheat

Wheat is the third largest produced grain in the world today. Historians say wheat originated in Turkey in prehistoric times and was cultivated in the Middle East where it's popularity then spread to Europe. Corn originated in the New World, and rice in the Far East.

---

condroitin and throwing the painkiller drugs away, he joyfully rejoined a training program. This involved running hundred-yard dashes (10 of them in five minutes, at 63 years of age!). Although the knees were stiff and painful at first, they eventually became better and better.

It is unfortunate, though, that in today's medical environment, doctors absolutely insist that the weaker and more inflamed your joints become, the more you must avoid exercise. Then, your only options are inactivity, NSAIDS, walkers/wheelchairs or joint replacement surgery. All of which will not remove the underlying cause of your arthritis and cause increased discomfort and susceptibility to pain, swelling and the onset of other related conditions.

Want to make your joints stronger? Work out! Jog, run, walk, bike, take a step class — start off slow and build up your endurance. You've got to move those joints and ligaments.

PLANTAR FASCIITIS

After completion of this manuscript and, while it was being edited, Dr Schep was training with the rugby team. One evening he caught a thrown ball and started to run flat out for the score line. All of a sudden there was a sharp pain in his right foot and he had to stop and hobble off the field. He was almost crippled and could no longer train. For weeks, every time he tried to run, immediately there was this extremely severe pain in his foot. Every morning when he woke up, the pain in the foot was so severe he had to stretch and exercise it in order to even get down the staircase. He was very upset and wondered if he ever could run again.

A quick search of literature showed that thousands of people are disabled by plantar fasciitis, which is an inflammation of the muscle tendons and ligaments that join the heel bone to the foot bones. He read Internet reports posted by dozens of people who for years had tried everything, without success, in hope of finding a cure. Some eventually resorted to wheelchairs. He also noted the devastating psychological feelings expressed by people in the reports and the sadness that they could no longer walk.

Dr. Schep knew he was now challenged to prove everything he had written in this chapter and that the challenge was to cure himself. He wondered how his feet (that he took for granted) had stood up to 50 years of tremendous pounding and running only to have problems now?

He found Web sites that wanted to sell all kinds of gadgets and solutions. From splints to place your foot into when you sleep at night to prolotherapy, an expensive system of injecting all kinds of irritants in the foot muscle. Finally, after weeks of searching, a tremendous breakthrough. He found a publication that indicated the material, which joins the foot tendon to the ankle bone, is nothing other than — cartilage. The same material inside our joints that protects the bones against pounding during running and walking. In a flash, he knew the cure — it was nutritional! It wasn't all of the many gadgets and gizmos, painkillers and prolotherapy. He also knew it takes three months to "heel" broken bones, so he instituted a three-month plan to start playing again. The regime was as follows:

2,500 milligrams vitamin C a day (accelerates healing of collagen and cartilage).

5 capsules omega-3 oil (prevents inflammation).

5 capsules glucosamine chondroitin sulfate (promotes healing of cartilage).

Weekly ultrasound treatments (increases circulation). (Person must be trained in the use of ultrasound, such as a chiropractor.)

4 milligrams of copper per day (increases SOD inside cells, lessening inflammation).

Optional: Ginger capsules 3 to 5 and bromelain capsules, 3 to 5.

Although Dr. Schep did not encounter this remedy anywhere, weekly he ate clams and oysters, taking special attention to scrape off the tough rubbery little "foot" of the clam or oyster where it is attached to the shell, and eat it. (The clam uses this "foot" to clam shut and protect itself from being eaten.)

After about four weeks, Dr. Schep suddenly got diarrhea. This meant his body had completed the healing from the vitamin C and his body did not want anymore vitamin C, so he discontinued it. (For persons with osteoporosis, this amount could be accepted by the body for years.) He continued with the rest of the treatment.

The plantars faciitis incident happened exactly three months before Christmas. The day after Christmas, Dr. Schep reported for rugby training. The foot was still tender and painful, but he could flat out run and the pain did not increase. He scored six points from kicking in the subsequent three months (Division I, 2010 session) and at the time of writing, the team is playing in the Western finals. If the team wins, they go on to national finals.

Dr. Schep continues to take the glucosamine chrondroitin sulfate. As you get older, the cartilage ages faster than the body can replace it and this supplement speeds up the formation of cartilage. Now, he thinks he made a mistake discontinuing the glucosamine years ago when he cured his arthritis. Had he not done that, he may not have had the plantar fasciitis problem.

GLUTEN ALLERGIES

About one in every 100 people has a severe reaction to gluten. While some people simply have a gluten allergy, many people have a condition named celiac disease, or celiac sprue. Celiac disease is when the intestines are so inflamed they cannot properly absorb nutrients. This means that even if you are consuming a diet rich with vitamins and nutrients, your body ceases the ability to use them.

Celiac disease is a digestive disease that damages the small intestine and interferes with the absorption of nutrients from food. When people with celiac disease eat food containing wheat, rye, barley and maybe oats, the person's immune system is triggered and inflammation results. This causes the immune system to damage the villi in the lining of the small intestine. The function of the villi is to absorb nutrients from the food. Unless the villi function properly, a person can become malnourished. So even if you are eating a lot of food and taking in healthy amounts of protein, minerals, vitamins and other vital elements, you actually could starve to death. The good news is that the villi are not permanently damaged and the intestine can heal itself, if the damage is solely due to celiac disease.

Anyone with a gluten allergy or diagnosed with celiac sprue should avoid all consumption of wheat, rye, barley and spelt. In other words, all grain from the *Tricticum* family must be avoided. *Tricticum* is the botanical genus name for wheat, of which there are about 14 different types of wheats/grasses. Because gluten allergy is in part a wheat allergy, this family must be avoided.

Some people also may be allergic to oat gluten, so oat products should also be avoided.

It is important to know when dealing with gluten allergies that wheat, rye and barley are related. Oats and rice are in the same subfamily as wheat, but in a different "tribe."

GRAIN FAMILY RELATIONSHIPS

The following is a ranking of grains; the lowest being the least related to wheat:

Wheat
Rye
Barley
Oats
Rice
Cane sugar
Millet
Corn

Wheat, rye, spelt, barley and possibly oats have a protein in them called gluten. Gluten contains a protein called gliadin. A clinical laboratory can perform a test called an antigliadin test (AGA) to find out if you have antibodies to gliadin in your blood. About one in five people have gliadin antibodies in their body. This is a large percentage of people. If you do have antibodies to gliadin, then you are allergic to wheat, rye and barley. Most people who have antibodies to gliadin do not notice any health affects, but it in some people the effects can be quite severe, including:

Bloating

Gas

Diarrhea

Constipation

Rectal itch

Osteoporosis

Nervous disorders (even Schizophrenia)

Fatigue

Depression

Skin problems

Itchy skin sensations

Arthritis

Substituting gluten-rich products with gluten-free products may seem daunting at first. But once you get the hang of it, you'll be happier, healthier and more satisfied as gluten-free foods tend to be more dense and filling. When recipes call for wheat, rye or barley, try using rice, buckwheat, corn, millet or quinoa. The latter is not even a grass, it is from the spinach family. Rice flours used for baking also taste really good.

Processed foods may contain hidden amounts of gluten, especially if processed in a plant that makes other items. If you eat prepackaged foods and snacks, make sure you read all package labels and nutritional labels. If you have severe gluten allergy, the slightest amount of gluten could have negative effects on you and even jump start previously relegated inflammation.

Celiac patients can try to lessen this form of inflammation by taking omega-3, about three to four capsules a day. The omega-3 supports the production of anti-inflammatory substances in the body and should lessen the inflammation of the digestive system.

No painkillers, NSAIDS or any other over-the-counter or prescribed drugs for the relief of pain or inflammation, joint pain, headaches, colds or flu should be used, as this will aggravate the stomach and intestines for celiac patients.

The gold standard for proper diagnosis of celiac disease involves getting an intestinal biopsy. An invasive biopsy that may not be necessary if you had a positive result with just the antigliadin test (AGA). A positive result from either test will require you to eliminate gluten from your diet. The only reason you may want a biopsy is to medically confirm you have to eliminate wheat from your diet. Independent of any test, try removing gluten from your diet and see what happens. You might notice a really positive change in your regularity, stomach condition and energy level.

In our section on life extension and anti-aging, we are going to show that excessive carbohydrates shorten lifespan and increase heart disease, cancer and diabetes. All grains, including wheat, supply carbohydrates to the diet.

FOODS CONTAINING GLUTEN

Many foods are hidden sources of gluten, namely some brands of the following products:

Soy sauce

Modified food starch

Ice cream

Soups

Beer

Vodka

Whiskey

Malts

As a matter of fact, any processed food has the potential of added gluten or contamination. You have to read labels!

There are various names used for wheat, rye, barley and other products. We've listed some foods to avoid:

Barley

Bulgur

Couscous

Dinkle

Durum

Einkorn

Emmet

Farina

Fu

Graham flour

Kamut

Matzo

Mir

Rye

Seiton

Semolina

Spelt

Cautionary measures should be applied to the following:

Bran

Oats

Edible starch

Malt

Any processed foods that may have hidden gluten

GRAINS AND FLOURS FOR A GLUTEN-FREE LIFESTYLE

Brown rice and flours

Almond flour

Arrowroot starch

Cassava

Coconut flour

Corn flour

Cornstarch

Flaxseed-meal

Millet

Tapioca

Quinoa

Sago

We have noticed that health and natural food stores sell packages of gluten-free flour mixes for making cake, pancakes, etc. Avoid the mixes where the first ingredient listed is white rice or any refined grain. We found one mix where sugar was listed as the first ingredient. No, no! These foods are lacking in minerals like iron, zinc and copper.

VITAMIN A TO THE RESCUE

In no other system of cure, except in this book, will you find the recommendation to use vitamin A to help improve digestive tract health or make it more resistant to gluten ingestion. Vitamin A helps the formation of cells that make mucous and is an important factor in the health of the mucous membranes. In other words, it will accelerate the healing of the villi. It also will make the villi less susceptible to gluten damage as new mucous cells will grow quicker to replace damaged ones. The more mucous formed, the easier it is to remove toxic and indigestible substances from the mucous membranes. Vitamin A also improves eye sight — better to read those labels, and avoid gluten.

The highest vitamin A content in carotene form is *red palm oil*, but sweet potatoes, carrots, kale, spinach, winter squash and mangos also are great sources.

Because of the trace mineral copper deficiency being the "silent unknown" cause of heart disease and cancer and, because it is lacking in the food produced by the American industrialized agricultural system, we have become suspicious as to whether it may also be the cause of gluten intolerance and celiac disease. No scientific papers on celiac versus copper deficiency could be found however. But the following facts emerge:

Roy Jamron reports the case where only one of identical twins got celiac.

In India, it is reported that only 1 in 310 children get celiac disease as opposed to the U.S. where it is 1 in 100.

The United States has much more industrialized agriculture, which produces copper-deficient food.

A Mayo Clinic study tested blood samples from male Army volunteers from 1948 to 1954. The study found that young people today have a 4.5 times higher rate of having the celiac antibody than during the years of study.

Dr. Klevay has reported a steady decline in copper in our food since the 1920s[20]. In 2003, Joseph Murray and associates[33] found celiac nine times higher in people than a decade ago. He said, "Something has changed in our environments to make it more common." (The increase of large amounts of corn syrup in our processed foods would decrease the copper content of our food.)

The common and accepted scientific argument — celiac disease is hereditary — does not fit these facts. The fact that our diets have increasingly less copper does fit these facts. Therefore, it is recommended that those with gluten intolerance and celiac disease increase their copper and other trace elements intake by eliminating sugar and foods containing corn syrup from their diet. They also should adopt the adequate copper diet to get at least 2 to 4 milligrams of copper per day.

Even if copper deficiency does not cause gluten intolerance, improving the copper intake will overcome impaired copper absorption by the gut, which will protect against heart disease and cancer.

Are you wondering what you can eat on a gluten free diet? Here are some ideas that will keep you on the right track and help make you feel satisfied:

Fruits and vegetables (unpackaged, fresh)

Meats (unseasoned)

Poultry and fish (unseasoned)

Grains (check the label, there only should be one ingredient and it should not say "contains wheat")

Cereal (buy specialty gluten-free cereals or Rice or Corn Chex)

Eggs (make scrambled eggs, frittatas, omelets, etc.)

Salads (add lean meat, cheese or chickpeas for added flavor and protein)

Wraps (use sliced meat instead of a tortilla to wrap cream cheese or hummus and vegetables)

Rice

Quinoa

Corn

Tapioca

Buckwheat

Soybeans

Carob

Arrowroot

Millet

If you are really struggling and you just have to have a brownie, a cookie or something that looks, tastes and feels like bread, there are many gluten-free products available at mainstream grocery stores. Betty Crocker® even has a line of gluten-free desert mixes that are really delicious. You also can find some great gluten-free cookbooks in bookstores and

Fast Facts

According to an article written by Eric Margolis and published in the Toronto Sun, "Americans, who comprise only 5 percent of the world's population, account for a whopping 33 percent of total global sugar consumption — over 10 million tons annually."

there are a lot of online recipes as well. We are sure you will feel full, satisfied and much healthier once you remove the gluten from your diet.

Even if you do not suffer from celiac disease or other gluten allergies, you might be wondering after reading this section what you can eat to lose weight and feel great. In addition to the delicious array of recipes you will find in Chapter 10, we've listed (at left) some of the best anti-cancer foods to eat and their benefits.

HIGH IN COPPER AND MANGANESE
Liver, oysters, dark chocolate, cashew nuts, sesame seeds, almonds, blackstrap molasses and oat bran.

HIGH IN SELENIUM
Brazil nuts.

HIGH IN VITAMIN C
Acerola cherry, guava, bell peppers, kiwifruit, and papaya.

HIGH IN OMEGA-3 AND OMEGA-9
Wild salmon, olive oil, safflower oil, and chia seeds.

HIGH IN VITAMIN D
Salmon (sockeye), sardines, shrimp, milk, cod and eggs.

IMMUNE BOOSTER
Mushrooms and strawberries.

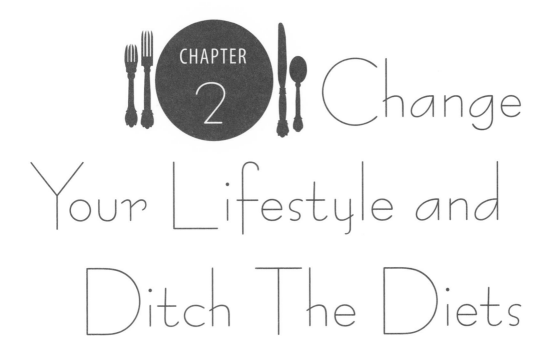

CHAPTER 2

Change Your Lifestyle and Ditch The Diets

Processed food and fast-food makers are deliberately putting substances into the foods they make. By adding substances that artificially stimulate your appetite, you can become addicted, and the net result is an addiction that can make you obese and shorten your life.

We are here to help you learn the truth about processesd foods, appetite suppressants and about the harm excess carbohydrate intake wreaks on your body. We will show you that you can eat as much as you need to satisfy your hunger, prevent obesity, and increase your life span, allowing more beautiful sunrises in your lifetime.

Protein, not diet pills or packaged diet food plans, is the true natural appetite satisfier. Eating protein in the morning satisfies your appetite for the entire day, which will lead to a decreased caloric intake all day long without making you feel hungry. If you are overweight, you will learn how to easily and rapidly bring your weight to a normal range without subjecting yourself to frustrating fad diets and stomach operations, instead, simply by eating differently.

Calories from carbohydrate-laden foods can decrease your life span. High levels of carbohydrates in you diet increases blood glucose levels causing inflammation in the body, makes you fat, causes diabetes and is damaging to your joints. (Fat does not contain glucose and does not elevate blood glucose levels as much as carbohydrates.)

Join us on this journey. You will feel good making these changes.

"BIG FOOD": THE PROCESSED FOOD INDUSTRY

Have you ever been low on dog or cat food and to get by until you could run to the store the next day you made them a nice big bowl of grits, plain rice or potatoes? We have, and you can be sure our pets turned their noses up in disgust. Who can blame them, right? However, when we poured a nice, flavorful gravy packet or added some shredded luncheon meat to the mix, they rushed right back and wolfed the whole thing down like it was a rare delicacy and then came to us looking for more.

The sad thing is, the food processing industry and chain restaurant corporations are doing the same thing to us! They take cheap, low quality, un-nutritious foods and add sauces, seasonings and fats to make it delicious. Even worse, they add substances to the food to make it addictive.

Umami (Flavor)

Over a hundred years ago, a Japanese doctor, Dr. Kikunae Ikeda, wondered why kombu (kelp) was so attractive in Japanese cooking, particularly in stocks and soups. After analyzing the kelp, he found that it contained an amino acid called glutamic acid (monosodium glutamate (MSG) is the salt of glutamic acid). After his research, he discovered that there was a fifth primary taste in our taste buds (after sweet, sour, salt and bitter). He called this taste *umami*, or flavor.

Dr. Ikeda found that glutamic acid had a strong umami factor and that people re-

Fact

Americans consume over 4.3 BILLION POUNDS of snack foods (chips, crackers, popcorn, etc.)!

sponded to and craved that taste in their foods. Since then, more compounds like inosinate and guanylate have been found to produce the same taste and response. These ingredients are used today in things like Worcestershire® Sauce. Have you ever looked at the ingredients list on a bag of Cheetos®? You'll find glutamate fairly close to the beginning of the ingredients list. That yellowish/orange color doesn't even come from carotenes or corn — it is a lifeless, artificial food coloring with no nutritional value whatsoever! The flavoring in Cheetos comes from MSG, which is added to corn. In its own right, kombu is rich with minerals and iodine. However, the MSG that is added to corn to flavor snacks like Cheetos and other chips, holds little (or none) of the original mineral or nutritional value.

Currently, the worldwide production amount of monosodium glutamate is unclear. However, Vietnam can produce 120,000 metric tons per year and other countries could be producing several times that amount.

Casein

Casein is a protein substance that occurs naturally in milk and can also be found in the seeds of leguminous plants. Unfortunately, "Big Food" has found a way to refine it, concentrate it, strip the nutrition out of it and then use it as an ingredient to help thicken or bind foods. Cheese makers remove the water, lactose and whey proteins (all the good stuff) from the casein to make a concentrated version.

Research has shown that the peptides in casein actually are addictive — similar in a way as morphine and heroin. The peptides from casein react with the opiate receptors in the brain, mimicking the effects of heroin and morphine. Numerous processed foods contain casein, including, but not limited to:

Sausages

Soups, stews

High protein beverage powders

Fortified cereals

Infant formula

Nutrition bars

And the list just goes on. The short story? By adding casein to these foods, the manufacturers are addicting you to their foods and creating more demand for the products. This equals higher profits for the industry, but even higher risks to your health.

Ireland is a big producer of casein, and the farmers there are subsidized by the government. It is very similar to what the sugar cane industry is doing: extracting the sucrose from the sugar cane, concentrating it and making it super sweet — addicting you to the sweetness.

Although flavorings and addictive agents in processed food and fast foods may play a role in obesity, in our own experiences, we have found that high-quality protein is the best true natural appetite satisfier. We have also learned (the hard way) that high carbohydrate/low protein foods do not satisfy our appetite, causing us to eat still more carbohydrates, sugars and fats.

WEIGHT CONTROL

Why should we be concerned about our weight? Because weight control is not about physical appearance or body shape, it is about heart disease, cancer, diabetes, arthritis, infectious diseases and a shortened life span.

When you are overweight, it indicates that you may have a problem with high blood sugar, which is harmful to the body causing: aging of the body, inflammation and damaged joints

The joint damage is not so much caused by excess weight resting on the joints (as we discussed earlier, healthy joints can take immense punishment), but by high blood sugar, which inflames the joints in particular but also the body as a whole.

A High Carbohydrate Diet Can Kill You

Ingesting a regular diet high in carbohydrates does incredible damage to your body, including causing arthritis, heart disease, diabetes, cancer, inability to fight infection and shortening your life span. About 20 years ago, surprising results of a study were announced. Rats or mice who were given access to food for 24 hours a day had much shorter life spans than those rats and mice who were only allowed to eat three times per day and whose food was removed after meal time. The rats that had food only three times a day lived 50 percent longer than the animals with unrestricted 24-hour access to food. At first there was no explanation for this but, soon, over the years, understanding the reason became clear. The excess calories and empty carbohydrates were the cause of the drastic life span difference between the two test groups.

The following information from a publication by The Life Extension Foundation, illustrates the harm and shortened life span caused by excess calorie and carbohydrate intake.

Caloric restriction is the most effective and well-documented pathway to longevity in animal studies. Both the mean and maximum life spans of yeast, rotifers, water fleas, nematodes, fruit flies, spiders, fish, hamsters, rats, mice and dogs have been extended significantly by decreasing normal caloric consumption by 30 percent to 40 percent (R. Weindruch[34], 1988). When caloric restriction with optimal nutrition (CRON) is begun in young animals, they remain smaller and leaner than their free-feeding counterparts. They also withstand a number of stressors better than their free-feeding counterparts (Berg T.F.[35], 1994; Heydari A.R.[36], 1993).

Young rodents consuming 40 percent fewer calories than their free-feeding counterparts generally will experience about a 50 percent increase in their life spans. Regardless of when CRON is started, its benefits appear to be proportional to both the degree and duration of caloric restriction (Merry B.J.[37], 2002). Thus, health benefits might be expected even when CRON is started late in life (Rae M., 2004). Since the longevity response to CRON appears to be conserved across the animal kingdom, primates and humans will likely benefit from CRON as well.

Merry's[37] publication seems pretty profound because he stated that superoxide production in the mitochondria (nucleus of the cell and the factory of the body) of the short-lived, unrestricted, fed animals was higher. So copper also may surface as an anti-aging ingredient as it increases superoxide dismutase that neutralizes superoxide.

Caloric Restriction With Optimal Nutrition (CRON) in Primates and Humans

The National Institute on Aging (NIA), the University of Wisconsin and the University of Maryland are currently conducting caloric restriction with optimal nutrition (CRON) studies on primates. Statistically, significant differences in longevity will not be available until 2010, but preliminary results are encouraging. In the NIA study, the number of deaths in the CRON group is approximately half that of those fed at will. For example, only 33 percent of the CRON squirrel monkeys have died compared with 54 percent of the free-feeding controls. For rhesus monkeys, so far, mortality is 13 percent for the CRON group and 23 percent for the free-feeding group (Lane MA et al, 2002). So the CRON longevity trends are in a positive direction. As of July 2009, 80 percent of the restricted calorie monkeys are alive, *half of the unrestricted calorie* monkeys are dead.

The New York Times article of July 9, 2009, shows a photo (at present, Internet accessible, *http://www.nytimes. com/2009/07/10/science/10aging.html*) of two of the rhesus monkeys, Canto and Owen. Canto, 27, who consumed the low-calorie diet, looks young, muscular, alert and fit; and Canto, 29, who received the high-calorie diet, is stooped, wrinkled and flabby.

Although life-span CRON studies have not been conducted on humans, there is anecdotal evidence and short-term data to suggest that CRON might work in humans as well. For example, the island of Okinawa has up to 40 times as many centenarians as does the rest of Japan. The caloric intake of adult Okinawans is 20 percent lower than their mainland counterparts. Children in Okinawa consume only about 60 percent of the recommended intake of food as their mainland counterparts (Bradley J. Wilcox[38]). The longevity of this subpopulation may be because of their restricted diet, although other factors cannot be ruled out.

Similarly, data from the Baltimore Longitudinal Study of Aging suggests that long-lived humans exhibit some of the same physiological and biochemical changes that accompany caloric restriction in animals. Survival rates are highest in those with low body temperatures and low levels of circulating insulin (Roth G. S.[39], 2002). In addition, levels of serum dehydroepiandrosterone (DHEA), a presumed longevity marker, are also higher in long-lived individuals (Kalimi M.[40] et al, 1999).

How Does CRON Promote Longevity?
Because caloric restriction decreases body weight, especially dangerous abdominal fat, researchers originally thought its ability to prolong life was associated with decreased fat.

However, this hypothesis was questioned after a study showed that genetically obese Zucker rats experienced no change in body fat percentage while on CRON compared to free-feeding controls, even though the restricted animals weighed less (Harrison D. E.[41], 1984). Mounting evidence suggests that CRON acts, at least in part, by improving insulin sensitivity, thereby reducing insulin and glucose levels.

The data suggest that most people consume too many calories for optimal health. Part of the problem may be evolutionary. Stone Age humans consumed few calories from simple carbohydrates (sugars) and more from complex carbohydrates (starch), which are rich in natural fiber. High-fiber foods tend to be more filling than simple refined sugars and refined carbohydrates such as white flour.

The establishment of agriculture about 10,000 years ago (Eaton S.B.[42], 1997) dramatically changed the nature of the human food supply. Carbohydrate-rich grains became available in large quantities. Then, in the past century, the grains were stripped of their fiber by processing, resulting in a steady dietary supply of refined carbohydrates. These refined carbohydrates are a dense source of calories, although not a great source of nutrition.

People who live in North America are advised to eat no more than about 55 percent of their calories as carbohydrates (Anderson J. W.[43], 1994), but not refined sugar and grains that are depleted of fiber. By relying on complex carbohydrates and dramatically reducing intake of calories, CRON produces dramatic weight loss, which improves insulin sensitivity and insulin action. It is worth noting, too, that the CRON animal studies generally have shown that CRON counteracts aging and prevents the diseases of aging regardless of the composition of the diet, if adequate nutrients are consumed.

Caloric Restriction in Today's World
Even if our genes still lived in the Stone Age, we do not. To maximize our longevity, we need to find a way to have the benefits of caloric restriction without being constantly distracted by hunger. One of the persistent problems with people and CRON is low compliance. Maintaining a dramatically reduced caloric intake over the long-term can be very demanding, especially in a culture surrounded by inexpensive, plentiful, calorie-rich, nutrient-poor food. Realistically, few people are willing to reduce their caloric consumption by 30 percent to 40 percent.

Two approaches are currently being explored to make the benefits of CRON more accessible. The first is the most direct: reducing calories by 30 percent to 40 percent. This requires a careful diet that is rich in nutrients, complex carbohydrates, soluble fiber and lean protein. Soluble fiber has been shown to decrease hunger, although hunger cannot realistically be eliminated completely during a dedicated CRON diet. Consuming fiber before meals can reduce the rapid absorption of simple carbohydrates and help decrease the post-meal surge in insulin (Anderson J.W.[44] et al, 1993).

Risk of Type 2 Diabetes

The relationship between insulin and diabetes (and heart disease) is well established. Insulin is a critical hormone that enables the transport of blood sugar (glucose) into our cells, where it is used to generate energy. As people age, their cells become resistant to insulin, a condition called insulin resistance. In response, blood levels of insulin rise, along with blood levels of glucose. This condition of elevated glucose and insulin is a major risk factor for type 2 diabetes. CRON not only prevents these changes, but can substantially reverse them. In fact, some researchers believe that CRON's ability to extend life span is related to its ability to modulate insulin and glucose levels.

In rats, CRON significantly reduces fasting and after-meal glucose levels by 10 to 20 percent, and reduces plasma insulin by about 50 percent (Kalant N.[45], 2001). This also is true in primates (Lane M. A.[46], 1999). (The inhabitants of Biosphere 2 experienced a 20 percent drop in blood sugar.) Decreases in plasma insulin and glucose can be observed even after one month of 10 percent restriction in primates, before any weight loss has occurred (Lane M.[47], 2001).

High Calorie Intake Causes Oxidative Damage to the Body

In addition to lowering risk factors for cardiovascular disease and diabetes, animals on CRON exhibit less oxidative damage than their free-feeding counterparts. Oxidative damage is caused by *reactive oxygen species* (ROS), such as the superoxide or "burning oxygen molecule," which causes serious damage within cells and cell membranes.

CRON counters this free-radical damage by accelerating the repair of damaged cell structures and making cell membranes more resistant to ROS. Consequently, some researchers believe caloric restriction to be "the most effective modulator of free radical-induced oxidative stress (Yu B.P.[48,49]).

CRONs Beneficial Effects on Cells

CRON reduces the cellular damage that is typically associated with unrestricted diets, including accumulation of ROS products, lipid peroxidation, (means fats becoming rancid), oxidized proteins and other measures of cellular aging (Dubey A.[50], 1996).

CRON Protects Cells

CRON increases the ability of the body to defend against ROS damage in other ways. In fruit flies and rodents following CRON, the levels of internal anti-oxidant enzymes, such as superoxide dismutase and catalase, are protected from age-related decline (Lin Y.J.[51] et al, 1998).

Aging rats on CRON have an anti-oxidant capacity comparable to that of younger animals. This is partly because of elevated levels of glutathione, a powerful internal anti-oxidant (Armeni T.[52], 1998).

Cancer-Limiting Effects of CRON

The anti-tumor effects of caloric restriction are well documented in experimental animals, and epidemiological studies in humans suggest a protective effect. CRON protects rats and mice from both spontaneous tumors and tumors induced by carcinogenic chemicals or radiation (Weindruch R.[53], 1988).

Studies show that: Breast cancer tumors (which developed after two months in laboratory rats who were administered a carcinogen) stopped growing when the rodents were put on CRON (Kritchevsky, D.[54], 1984).

Excess Carbohydrate's Damage to the Body (Glycation)

So how does excess carbohydrate shorten the life span of animals? It is called glycation. Carbohydrates cause blood glucose to rise and this is extremely damaging to the body. How does glucose damage the body? By a process called glycation.

What is glycation? In each of our bodies we have protein molecules. Glucose and aldehydes from the body attach themselves to those protein molecules and become like a piggy-back rider on the molecule. When the molecule with the rider comes into contact with another protein molecule, the rider grabs the new protein by a process called cross-linking. As our body is made up almost entirely of protein, and cross-linking can happen easily and rapidly, the glycation process can cause severe problems, such as:

Decreased brain function because of glycated protein in the brain (associated with Alzheimer's).

Skin wrinkling (for some, this is the worst symptom of all!).

Hardened veins and arteries.

Difficulty in insulin passing from the blood into cells (insulin resistant diabetes).

Shortening of life span, as much as 50 percent in animal studies.

Altered proteins put the immune system on alert, causing the immune system to attack the glycated proteins as foreign material This causes inflammation in the body, associated with heart disease, cancer and arthritis. It is similar to putting a stick into the spokes of a bicycle wheel while it is moving.

So what substances cause glycation? It is sort of like a sliding scale, with different substances coming in at different percentages. The higher the starch value, the higher the glucose level and, coincidentally, the higher the carbohydrate level. Sugars are fructose-rich, while starch basically supplies only glucose. Some interesting facts:

Cane sugar (sucrose) is made up of 50 percent glucose and 50 percent fructose.

Fructose has 10 times the glycating ability of glucose.

High-fructose corn syrup number 55 (HFCS 55) is made up of 45 percent glucose and 55 percent fructose (meaning it is 8 percent more glycating than sugar).

Starch, being only glucose, has only 20 percent the glycating ability of sugar.

With sugar, the body has to break up the sucrose molecule into fructose and glucose. Even worse, the glucose and fructose in high-fructose corn syrup number 55 (sadly, a common ingredient in sports drinks, sodas, packaged foods and snacks, etc.) are in a free form and go straight into the blood stream, so the blood sugar concentration is higher and moves faster. Because of this, high-fructose corn syrup number 55 may have an even higher glycating percentage compared to sugar or sweeteners derived from sugar cane.

High-fructose corn syrup number 55 has overtaken the use of sugar in processed and prepackaged foods. The reason: It is cheap, easy to transport (it is a liquid and can be moved quickly and easily in large containers), and it's easy to use in manufacturing because it doesn't need to be dissolved in water to be made usable. High-fructose corn syrup number 55 is also subsidized by the government through subsidies to corn farmers. The bottom line? The government is using your own money to destroy your health to keep costs down and corn farms in the black.

The good news — The following substances act as anti-glycating agents.

Resveratrol: The red color in wine and an anti-glycating and anti-aging agent.

Carnosine: A peptide (made in the body from the amino acids beta-alanine and histidine). Carnosine prevents protein molecules from sticking together, eliminating the issue of cross-linking. Carnosine is found in meat (particularly beef, poultry and pork), eggs and cheese.

Enjoy bagels or croissants for breakfast? Add a nice thick slice of ham and an egg and/or a glass of milk to help counteract the glycation process.

For dinner, enjoy grilled chicken breast with steamed vegetables and brown rice with a nice glass of red wine. Not only is this meal low in calories, low in fat, low in sugar and carbohydrates and delicious, it is high in nutrients, minerals and anti-glycating agents. Not to mention good for your skin!

So how does this information relate to you and your weight? It's simple. Being overweight comes from too many calories, not faulty metabolism, stress or other outside factors.

We all know that calories are the body's fuel, but if you take in more calories than your body needs, you will gain weight. You will especially gain weight if the excess calories you take in are in the form of carbohydrates, since carbohydrates turn into glucose, which plays with your blood sugar and protein molecules, as discussed above.

We all have either had our own weight struggles or know people who were/are struggling with their weight. Some people who are overweight tend to blame slow metabolism for their weight. They may claim that they eat very little but just don't stop gaining weight. While they may in fact be eating very little, it's WHAT they are eating that causes the damage. For example: pancakes dripping in syrup for breakfast, one sandwich with plenty of mayonnaise, mustard and meat for lunch, two candy bars and one cheeseburger with fries and a sugar-loaded milkshake may not be a lot of food, but the quality of the food and the calories and carbohydrates contained in that food are off the charts! A tall, active, muscular, healthy weight person would gain weight on that diet. Is it a lot of food? Not really. Is it nutritious, lean and healthy? No way! Fat does not reproduce on its own, it has to be ingested to get inside our bodies. If your weight is increasing or you are not losing weight, it means you are taking in more calories than you are burning.

The media has led people to believe that exercise is the cure-all for weight loss. While it does play a big part in obtaining and sustaining a healthy body inside and out, it won't affect your weight if you are taking in more calories and carbohydrates than you are burning. Did you know that the average candy bar is roughly 300 calories? It takes one hour of intense exercise to burn that many calories, and then you'll just break you even. Bottom line? Less calories (back away from the candy bar) and still get that hour of exercise and you will lose weight, lower your blood sugar, increase circulation to your brain and heart, lower your blood pressure, sleep better and feel great.

Diet pills are also another media favorite. You see television commercials, magazine ads, billboards, hear radio testimonials and watch infomercials for these products. These pills are not the answer! Many of the products claim that you can eat whatever you want and not gain weight if you take their pills. This is the reason that the diet pill industry is such a dangerous, fraudulent industry. No matter what pills you take or how little or how much you eat, if you take in more calories than you burn, you will gain weight! Most diet pills are filled with substances that are completely unnatural too, causing such things as acne, headache, diarrhea, nausea, forgetfulness and other detrimental side effects. Diet pills are money-makers for the pill companies — They are not your quick-fix miracle.

To successfully lose weight and improve body function, you must understand that the major cause of obesity and life threatening inflammation and sugar and/or carbohydrate poisoning is due to excess consumption.

The process works like this:

The carbohydrates we take in (breads, pasta, pastries, etc.) are converted into glucose, which goes into the blood stream. If you take in more carbohydrates than your body needs (which most of us do on a daily basis), the body causes the blood glucose levels to rise. The glucose then combines with the proteins in the body and the glycation process begins (as discussed above). Once the glycation process has occurred, the glycated proteins put the immune system on alert (like an SOS — foreign substances are here, attack!). The immune system then attacks these proteins, because it sees them as degraded or foreign materials threatening the body. This causes inflammation. In simpler terms, if the protein, cartilage and ligaments in our joints become glycated, our immune system attacks them, causing inflammation and pain.

PROTEIN IS A SUPER FOOD

The important nutritional information to remember — Protein is a super food. Protein does amazing things, such as:

Replenishes the body.

Builds and maintains muscles.

Strengthens bones by increasing collagen content.

Supplies energy to the body.

Supplies anti-aging substances.

Carbohydrates are a much more inferior food. While they do supply energy, the unused energy they contain converts to body fat. So, if you want to be lean, energized, healthy, have youthful looking skin and pain-free joints — Replace excess carbohydrates and increase the protein!

Protein Prevents Inflammation That Causes Aging

Animal protein is high-quality protein and it is a natural appetite suppressant. It is needed for muscles, tendons, ligaments and, yes, even bones, cartilage and joints. Protein makes *Tissue Inhibitor of Matrix Metalloproteinase* (TIMPS). TIMPS is a cysteine-containing polypeptide and cysteine blocks matrix metalloproteinase (MMP) receptors. TIMPS inhibits MMPs (Schütz R.[55] 2006), therefore protein is anti-inflammatory.

As we mentioned, MMP (matrix metalloproteinase) is a destroyer of protein and therefore a destroyer of joints and bones and muscle in the body. Matrix is just a fancy word for tissue. If the effect of MMPs are accented by a lack of omega-3s, high blood sugar from high carbohydrate intake and lack of protein (the typical American diet) the body is inflamed, joints are inflamed, the immune system is suppressed and you age. The compound cysteine is necessary to make TIMPS. Cysteine is in meats and fish, but soy is also a good source. Soy also contains genistin, which has been shown to fight breast cancer.

Some scientists claim that high levels of TIMPS in the body come with an increase in the rate of breast cancer. Soy, however, is known to lessen breast cancer (see Wu, A.[56] 1998). Soy contains cysteine and therefore will increase the level of TIMPS in the body. This means that the scientists are making an incorrect conclusion. They argue that the phytoestrogens (plant estrogens) in the soy could increase cancer. In the cancer section we show that estrogen does not cause cancer.

Genistin also increases TIMPs in the body and decreases MMPs. Heat destroys 20 to 50 percent of cysteine. Do not overcook your meat or your soy.

Vegetarians can take note that despite the fact that soy is a vegetable protein, it seems to protect you from inflammation.

Nutritional Value of Carbohydrates Versus Protein

The main function of carbohydrates in the body is to produce energy to be burned as calories. The calories that are not used are converted to fat and stored on your body. Carbohydrates (especially the simple ones [sugar]) while necessary for producing energy, are a concentrated form of glucose. They can cause blood glucose levels to rise very high very quickly, causing glycation, the precursor for inflammation. Also, unlike protein, carbohydrates do not have the ability to build muscle or strengthen bones. You have heard the term "empty calories" before, right?

Carbohydrates, especially when consumed as snacks, are nothing but empty calories. Hungry between meals? Back away from the pretzels and crackers! Grab a hard-boiled egg or wrap cream cheese or hummus in slices of lean luncheon meat. Protein, especially animal protein, is the perfect food because not only does it build muscles and strengthen bones, it also provides long-lasting energy and will leave you feeling satisfied far longer than any carbohydrate.

A high protein meal or snack is delicious, healthy, filling and helps keep your muscles and joints free of inflammation. Coincidently, high protein snacks are MUCH cheaper than carbohydrate snacks. For example, the average cost of one dozen eggs is about $1.50 and the average cost of eight ounces of lean luncheon meat from the deli counter is around $2.50. From one dozen eggs and eight ounces of meat you can easily make at least four days worth of snacks and breakfast. Here are some other great high protein, low carbohydrate meals and snacks:

Breakfast

    Two scrambled eggs wrapped in two slices lean deli meat.

    Two-egg omelet with sliced deli meat, sea salt and pepper.

    Two eggs sunny-side up on top of two slices lean deli meat.

    Two eggs scrambled with shredded deli meat.

Snack

    One hard-boiled egg.

    Two deviled egg halves (use sugarless mustard).

    Two deviled egg halves (mix in shredded deli meat).

    One scrambled egg wrapped in lean deli meat.

The bottom line? For approximately $4 (a dollar per day), which is *much less* than you would spend on carbohydrate-packed products like breads, muffins, toaster pastries, scones, etc., you can shrink your waistline, minimize inflammation in your joints, stave off muscle cramps, build your muscles, strengthen your bones and feel full and satisfied.

One dozen eggs: $1.50.

Eight ounces deli meat: $2.50.

Pain-free joints and a trim waistline: Priceless!

We know how hard it is to start reducing carbohydrates in your diets, but please believe us when we tell you how easy it becomes and how much better you'll feel. By replacing some of your daily carbohydrate intake with lean protein, you can limit glycation, stay or get lean and healthy and have a strong, fit body.

Another great benefit of animal or non-animal protein is that the liver takes the protein and turns it into glucose using a process called *glucogenesis*. Glucogenesis is the process of making energy from protein instead of carbohydrates. This can better regulate blood sugar and does not cause spikes. When blood sugar spikes occur, the body quickly uses what it needs and sloughs off the extra glucose, which attaches itself to the internal walls. The extra glucose then converts into fat and becomes a permanent fixture on our bodies. So by eating more protein and less carbohydrates, we can stop glycation, utilize glucogenesis and avoid adding fat to our bodies. You also will feel more energized, lighter and happier, and you won't suffer from as many mood swings or pre-menstrual symptoms. All of which are greatly affected by blood sugar spikes or irregular blood sugar levels. Protein, on the other hand, is regulated and does not cause high blood sugar.

We would like to take this opportunity to point out the difference between caloric restriction and the correction of the diet. If you read articles about prolonging your life in books, magazines, on the Internet and/or other media sources, you will see that many of the sources focus on calorie restriction. The truth is: Calories only damage our bodies when we take in more than our daily requirement.

In our attempts to diet while managing our busy lives, it is really easy to "take advantage" of the readily available, store-bought, prepackaged diet foods that are lined on the store shelves. These actually may be carbohydrate-based. Take a minute to reflect on either the last time you went on a diet to restrict calories or the last time you were at the grocery store. Do you remember what diet products you saw? We are guessing (from our own experiences) that you either saw or purchased some of these similar items:

Diet shakes or meal replacement bars.

Frozen diet meals (these are mostly pasta-based with added starches like potatoes).

Reduced-fat crackers or pretzels.

Pre-packaged diet cookies or snacks.

Low-fat soups (also, mostly pasta-based).

Before reading the previous information we've shared, you probably thought these were great options for the dieter on the go. Easy, convenient and, for the most part, filling. Right? Wrong! After the excitement of the new diet has worn off, do you feel yourself getting hungry between meals? Thinking about food after dinner? Wandering into the kitchen and aimlessly opening cupboard doors and the refrigerator? This is because 90 percent or more of the foods and snacks listed above are carbohydrate-based. So while they give you an initial sense of fulfillment and energy, they also take you on a dangerous "sugar low" when your body is looking for more energy to finish the day. But your body has already stored the great amount of extra carbohydrates, which it found unnecessary due to the initial spike in blood sugar. This means that you added more fat to your body, but you're still hungry and unsatisfied. Those feelings lead you back to the unhealthy habits you had before, adding even more inches to your waistline and inflammation to your joints. And that makes you feel sad and irritable at the "failure" of your diet. The good news? You don't need to subject yourself to that vicious cycle anymore!

Instead of dieting by restricting your calorie intake, start replacing your high carbohydrate, low protein foods with high protein, low carbohydrate foods. No, we don't mean radically cutting out all carbohydrates, expelling fruit and dairy from your diet and never having a cookie or sandwich again. Making just a few easy substitutions a few days a week is a great way to get started.

Here are some easy, delicious high-protein solutions to substitute for some of your regular carbohydrate intake.

The real truth about calorie restriction is that carbohydrates only cause harm when you consume more calories than what you use and the calories come from refined carbohydrates that cause a rapid rise in blood sugar. Glycation can be lessened considerably by consuming starch instead of sugar or, even worse, corn syrup.

It is important to remember that the body does need a minimum requirement of calories to carry out all its functions and to provide energy for the muscles to perform. The number of calories you need to perform your daily functions can be determined using simple formulas based on your height, age gender, and current weight. You can find these formulas online (search calorie counters), or you can talk with your doctor about what a healthy weight would be for you and what daily calorie range is just right for you, whether your goal is to lose weight, gain muscle, maintain your current weight or even gain weight. One warning you must take seriously: Once you have burned up your excess fat, calorie restriction below your body's necessary level will cause muscle loss and joint damage due to the use of muscle for food, not to mention it causes your metabolism to slow down, which can slow or stop your weight loss. Slow, planned, healthy weight loss is not only better for your body, but easier to maintain for the long run.

There is so much advice on TV and in other types of media about dieting and weight loss. But the truth is, about 95 percent of it is nonsense — ploys to get you to part with your money by companies who care more about their bottom line than your bottom line and waistline.

You view weight-loss Web sites and infomercials claiming that there are good carbohydrates and bad carbohydrates and that good carbohydrates have a low glycemic index and that bad carbohydrates have high glycemic index. This information, while it sounds good (especially when pictures of delicious-looking prepared meals are circulating around your screen), is just a theory.

In truth, all carbohydrates are bad carbohydrates if you consume more than you require and will cause damaging levels of glucose in your blood. Just like calories, fat, sugar, etc., if you consume more than your body needs, the body will turn it into fat. Your body doesn't care what the glycemic index of the carbohydrate is, it will just do its job and turn it into fat if you take in more then you need.

Diet Correction Versus Exercise

You might think: What if I still eat low protein, high carbohydrate foods but I exercise a lot? I still need the carbohydrates to fuel me for my weight loss, right? Unless you are running a marathon every day, or working out for five to eight hours each day, exercise alone is not going to help.

HIGH CARBOHYDRATE/ LOW PROTEIN FOOD	LOW CARBOHYDRATE/ HIGH PROTEIN REPLACEMENT
Plain bagel with butter	Half rye or whole-wheat bagel with one tea spoon peanut butter.
Sandwich on white or wheat bread	Tortilla wrapped around cream cheese and sliced meat.
Spaghetti with marinara sauce	Cooked and shredded butternut squash (cooks just like spaghetti noodles) with olive oil and sun-dried tomatoes. Watch the olive oil, 1 ounce is 247 calories. However, as it has no carbohydrates it has a zero glycemic load.
Crackers	Hard-boiled eggs.
Cereal	Scrambled eggs.
Pretzels	Sliced raw vegetables with cream cheese dip or hummus.
Pancakes or waffles	Egg omelet with cheese and side of fruit.

While exercise plays a huge part of your overall health, wellness and weight, you cannot use it as a leveraging tool. For instance, you can't justify that the 300 calories you burned running on the treadmill for one hour counter-acts the effects of your bowl of white flour-based cereal for breakfast and the latte with flavoring you grabbed on the way to the gym. Most people burn about 300 calories per hour doing intense exercise (maybe 600 to a thousand per hour if you are a champion runner or professional athlete in training). That rate constitutes a loss of approximately one-half pound in three hours. You can consume a 300-calorie candy bar in 30 seconds. Is that 30 seconds worth three hours of intense exercise, just to break even? And we mean break even calorically. Not to mention the chemicals, blood sugar spikes, processed ingredients and other unnatural, unhealthy additives that wreak havoc on more important things than your weight — your heart, kidneys, liver, pancreas, brain and more.

Think about it this way: Our ancestors, whoever they may be, did not have 1-800 diet programs to deliver food to them. They didn't have diet shakes and meal replacement bars, they didn't have the glycemic index. What they did have is mineral-rich soil, high-fiber diets rich in healthy fruits and vegetables, lean meats and fish and plenty of daily exercise. Because of those benefits, they were lean and muscular and didn't suffer from diabetes, heart disease, liver poisoning, high cholesterol, etc. It's time to get back to basics and follow our fore-fathers' footsteps.

THE TRUTH AND SECRETS ABOUT WEIGHT LOSS

Two important rules to know and understand about losing weight: To maintain your current weight, consume only as many calories as you burn each day; to lose weight, consume less calories than you burn each day.

In reality, there is no other way to successfully maintain or lose weight and keep it off. You can resort to plastic surgery techniques such as tummy tucks, liposuction, lapbands, gastric bypass, etc. Not only are these procedures time intensive, painful, expensive and dangerous, they won't solve your problem! When doctors get $10,000 to $25,000 for a lap-band procedure, it's no wonder there is a billboard every mile on the freeway promoting it. It is also a sorry and dangerous excuse for being unable to change your bad eating habits to healthy eating habits. You easily can go back to your old eating patterns after the surgery, having gone through all the pain and expense to land right back where you started. Remember the rule: Consume only the calories you need.

We realize consuming only the calories you need can be difficult. In the past, you probably have been highly motivated and excited about following through with your restricted-calorie diet. You may have promised yourself that THIS time you will really stay on track and meet your goal for good. But then the hunger strikes. Hunger is a powerful force and it can bring down the strongest, most motivated person. So, what can you do this time to change your life and be happy and healthy? You must conquer the beast and eliminate hunger.

To do that you must satisfy or "suppress" (to coin a term from those dreaded weight loss commercials) your appetite. To satisfy your appetite, all you have to do is consume your daily requirement of quality protein. This can easily be done while limiting your carbohydrate and calorie intake. Yes, it is really that simple! Give your body what it needs and wants and it will do the rest.

The only true, natural and safe appetite suppressant is quality protein. And the real cause of hunger is a lack of protein. Hunger is the signal the body gives off when it is lacking and demanding protein. If your child is thirsty and crying for water, you wouldn't give him or her a sucker or candy bar, right? You would hand over a big glass of water. We have to give ourselves the same respect and give our bodies what it is asking for. The trick is knowing what we want. Just like becoming a new parent for the first time and learning what each of your baby's different cries mean, you need to learn to listen to your body's signals and cries and learn what they mean.

If your body is craving protein, why eat carbohydrates containing little protein when you are hungry? Again, hunger is your body crying for protein. Carbohydrates will not satisfy your hunger, meaning if you eat them when they are not what the body needs, they will convert to fat. What is the real cause of obesity? Trying to satisfy your hunger with carbohydrates, carbohydrates and more carbohydrates.

If you do not get enough protein and attempt to satisfy your hunger with carbohydrates, you will continue to be hungry no matter how many carbohydrates you consume.

You have heard the funny saying "Where's the beef?" The saying is funny, but it started as a real question because meals just aren't complete and the body just isn't healthy without protein. One of the best proteins, which contains elements better than any vitamin, pill, diet supplement or shake, is chicken. Chicken is lean, low fat, no carbohydrates and high in protein.

Now, protein doesn't necessarily have to be animal protein (although we do prefer it because it has no carbohydrates). It can come from tofu or other vegetarian or vegan sources as well. The important lessons to remember — reduce carbohydrates and increase protein. Chia seeds contain the same percentage of protein as meat. Also be aware that corn-fed beef (most of the beef we buy) has 30 percent more calories than grass-fed beef. Corn-fed beef also does not contain omega-3; grass-fed beef does. Cows evolved to eat grass, not cornmeal. Nevertheless, fat has no glycemic index, carbohydrates do.

How Do We Lose Weight?

As we discussed earlier, weight loss by exercise alone is impractical. With one hour of exercise only burning approximately 300 calories, burning approximately 1.4 ounces of fat, it would take roughly 12 hours of exercise to burn one pound of fat! Unless you have the time, money, energy and will to spend that much time exercising at an intense level, it would be easier on you and your body to just reduce your calorie intake by a few hundred, or even a few thousand, calories per day. Now, a few hundred or thousand calories sounds like an awful lot, but if you have a lot to lose, you might not realize how many calories you are ingesting every day.

We recommend following your regular eating routine for a few days and writing down the calorie value of everything you ingest, including: drinks, snacks, gum, breath mints, meals, etc. Then, average the total number of calories for all of the days by how many days you journaled. For example, if you took in 2,600 calories on Monday,

6,290 calories on Tuesday, 4,600 calories on Wednesday, and 2,988 calories on Thursday, that is a total of 16,478 calories over four days. Divide the total number of calories (16,478) by the number of days (4) and you get an average daily intake of 4,119.5 calories. Using simple calculators available for free on the Internet, determine how many calories per day your body needs to complete all of its functions. For most of us, that basic need is between 1,500 and 2,500 per day, well below 4,000 calories. The sad fact is that in today's society, consuming 4,000 calories or more has become normal, hence the dire need for the information in this book to be widespread and put to good use. If your calorie requirement is 2,000 calories per day, then you need 8,000 calories over four days (16,478 calories minus 8,000 is 8,478 excess calories, divided by 3,500 calories (the amount of calories needed to make one pound of fat) and you will gain 2.4 pounds of weight gain over four days. The main problem with a low-calorie diet by means of food restriction is that it not only causes hunger, it doesn't provide your body with the levels and amounts of nutrition your body needs.

Even if you are successful reaching your weight loss goals by carbohydrate restriction and exercising like crazy, when you go off the diet, you start taking in excess calories again and then your weight increases right up to where it was originally. Usually, we actually reach our previous weight and add a little extra, making the task of "dieting" again almost unbearable. Not only is this hard on our bodies, but our minds and spirits suffer as well. You can only take failure so many times until you start believing that your goals are unreachable. That is not a healthy pattern of thought.

A rare, but serious, problem that can occur with calorie or food restriction is the severe reduction of daily zinc intake. When zinc is severely restricted by low food intake, you lose your appetite because zinc is necessary for your body to process taste and other taste-related sensations. Without those sensations, the body does not want food, which can trigger serious eating disorders resulting in anorexia, starvation and even death.

The Best Way to Lose Weight
The best way to lose weight is to deal with the *cause* of being overweight. The cause, plain and simple, is food. High-carbohydrate, low-protein food provides only calories and does not satisfy your appetite, take way your hunger or lubricate and strengthen your muscles and bones.

The major cause of obesity in the United States is the common practice of eating the wrong types of food, following temporary fad diets, and not being able to determine which type of diet is best for the body. All due to the confusing array of information from the media. We have said it many times already, but we just can't stress the importance of this one truth: The cause of obesity is eating a diet high in calories and low in protein. The body wants and asks for adequate protein. Therefore, the body is going to keep you hungry until you get enough

Note

Some farmers use the cheaper arsenic instead of antibiotics to make their chickens grow faster. Avoid this type and use bona fide organic chicken, available from many local farms, health food grocery stores, CSAs or farmers markets. Recently, some major supermarkets have added organic chickens to their selections.

protein (you know, that unsatisfied feeling you have right after you eat a big dinner that sends you scavenging around the kitchen even though you KNOW you shouldn't be hungry, but you just need something, anything, to eat?).

If you respond to the hunger (see scenario above) by eating more calories, the end result is increasing amounts of fat being stored in the body. This is NOT what we want, right? The solution is: If you are overweight, take in high protein low calorie food. Adequate protein satisfies the hunger and cuts off your body's hunger signals. That means you have no more desire for food, meaning no mindless snacking, no high sugar and carbohydrate deserts; and no feelings of guilt, irritation or anger at yourself. Why? Because you will feel full and satisfied!

The amazing result of getting enough protein and limiting your carbohydrates is that you will not be hungry and your body will get the adequate nutrition it craves. Once your body weight is within a normal range, you can take in your daily protein requirement plus whatever calories are needed for the day, and no excess.

In this way, you will maintain your healthy, lower weight the normal natural way, as well as correct the problem of trying to eliminate hunger by carb-loading. Sound too easy to be true? We assure you that it is, as we are living proof that this really works!

The First Step

The first step is to determine how many calories your body consumes in one day. For that you need a calorie calculator. There are many calorie calculators on the Web, as we discussed earlier.

The calorie counter should be used to help you find out how many calories you require per day. If you don't have access to the Internet or just aren't comfortable using the calorie counters you find online, you can use the following table to determine your approximate, appropriate daily calorie requirements.

The table below is based on a 50-year-old person that sleeps seven hours a day, reads, sits and works or watches TV for a combined time of 12 hours a day, and performs some light work involving standing and walking for about five hours a day.

With a high-protein diet, you may need less calories than this, as the body is capable of converting protein into glucose.

Females have a need for fewer calories but it is not because they have a different or slower metabolism. It is because a female with the same weight as a male normally will have less muscle and more fat than the male (sorry ladies), unless she is very slim or muscular. It is the muscles that utilize the calories more for energy and strength. The more muscle, the more calories can be taken in without impacting body weight.

Recommended Daily Calories

WEIGHT (IN POUNDS)	MALE	FEMALE
100	1,540	1,390
120	1,840	1,660
140	2,150	1,940
160	2,460	2,210
180	2,760	2,490
200	3,070	2,760

If you are overweight, you must try and change your diet so that you take in less calories per day than what you need and use. In this way, you will automatically lose weight without exercise, although exercise will be a great help in accelerating the weight loss and keeping you toned. (You don't want to be thin and saggy — thin and toned is much better!) Although exercise can be a slow way to lose weight, it does increase your muscle mass and ability. In turn, those muscles burn more calories, even when you are not exercising.

One pound of fat is the equivalent of 3,500 calories per day. So if you are overweight and, based on the proper calculations, your body requires 2,500 calories per day, change your diet to 1,500 calories per day. Your body will have to convert EXISTING body fat to 1,000 calories (energy) to make up the difference. This means that in three-and-one-half days your body will have converted one pound of fat into 3,500 energy units (calories) to burn and you will weigh one pound less! The best part — this process happens with little time and effort and it happens even while you are sleeping!

The formula can be calculated like this: Weight loss or gain in pounds: *Add* calories consumed *minus* calories used and *divide* by 3,500.

If the answer is a positive number, it is weight gain. If the answer is a negative number, it is weight lost.

The beauty of it all is that you can calculate and predict weight loss or gain as sure as you can calculate the balance in your checkbook.

The next step is to eat food equaling 1,200 calories a day and this can easily be achieved by eating high protein foods. The best high protein foods are animal proteins, but if you are a vegetarian or vegan you can substitute soy, beans and tofu.

Why High Protein Food?

The protein requirement for the body is one gram of protein for every kilogram of body weight, or 100 kilograms of protein for a or 220-pound person. The average weight of 150 pounds would require 68 grams of protein per day. Most of us only get about half that amount daily. This must change if we want to conquer obesity, lethargy and so many other medical and physical problems. We can do it — we just have to change our diets to contain foods that contain more protein and less carbohydrates.

Have you seen the people who are promoting a new diet plan called the "Negative Calorie Diet"? This diet company claims you can lose as much as two pounds per day. The company claims it works if you eat foods that use more calories to chew, digest, metabolize and eliminate than what you get from the food. The diet's recommended foods include celery, broccoli, carrots and others. The problem with the diet? It cannot be carried out indefinitely as it would cause muscle wasting.

Muscles, without the proper protein, vitamins and minerals (derived via the foods we eat) power the muscles, which power the entire body. On this diet, you would not get enough quality protein for your body and it certainly would not be suitable for sportive or athletic persons. Unless, of course, you are a chimpanzee in the jungle spending the whole day eating greens or grazing the whole day long like a cow and then chewing the cud at night! Plus, once you have lost all your extra weight, what are you going to eat?

The trick to long-term weight loss is to follow a program that is easy and effective and one that can be followed for the rest of your life without damaging your body, costing you a fortune or making you feel hungry and unsatisfied. The system we are teaching you works because you are going back to basics and listening to your body by eating a protein-adequate diet and eliminating excess calories naturally. And it can be done for the rest of your life, which, coincidentally, will be longer due to your decision to change the way you eat.

The low-calorie high-protein diet can and should be used until you reach a normal, healthy weight range for your body type, at which point you can then incorporate foods that give you enough calories to maintain your weight, and enough protein to maintain your body. This diet does incorporate "negative calorie" foods, but does not solely consist of them, it uses them to supply antioxidants and fiber to your body .

The next step is to eat a daily diet containing 1,500 calories a day. This can easily be achieved by eating high protein foods.

Animal Versus Vegetable Protein

So why do we promote animal protein over vegetable protein? There are two reasons:
1. Animal protein is the highest quality protein; vegetable protein is of lower quality.
2. Animal protein does not contain any carbohydrates and has fewer calories. Vegetable protein (corn, beans, grains, etc., are loaded with carbohydrate calories).

It is easy to get your daily protein requirement from animal protein without exceeding your calorie intake, but almost impossible to get your protein requirement from vegetable protein without exceeding your calorie requirement. (If you have concerns as a vegan or vegetarian, we will address those concerns later in this chapter).

The body digests protein and breaks it down into individual amino acids. Some amino acids can be made within the body, but others must be obtained from the foods that we eat. These amino acids are called *essential amino acids*. Animal protein contains, to a greater or lesser extent, all the essential amino acids that the body needs. This is not the case with vegetable protein. For example, corn has no or very little lysine, whereas, beans may have lysine but is low in methionine (lysine and methionine are essential amino acids derived from our diet).

Foods are rated according to the Protein Digestibility Corrected Amino Acid Score (PDCAAS). Protein quality is evaluated based on the amino acid requirements of humans. A PDCAAS value of 1 is the highest and zero (0) is the lowest. We've listed some PDCAAS ratings of common foods:

Eggs (1.0)
Casein (1.0)
Milk (1.0)
Whey (1.0)
Beef (0.92)
Kidney beans (0.68)
Lentils (0.52)
Peanuts (0.52)
Wheat (0.25)

> **Note**
>
> This formula calculates only the weight gain or loss in terms of body fat, so it is important to note that if you take in or lose a lot of water, this also will affect your weight. (This is why our body weight fluctuates daily, sometimes as much as two or three pounds per day).

You will see in the following table that animal protein is superior to vegetable protein in the sense that you can get your protein requirement easily without exceeding your calorie requirement. Specifically, eggs are an amazing wonder food because of the total level of nutrients contained (protein, vitamin A, etc.) and because of the perfect quality of the protein.

How do we lose weight easily, safely and healthily? Change our diet from high-carbohydrate low-protein to high-protein low-carbohydrate.

The food items listed in the following table start with those that have a high-protein content and a low-carbohydrate content. The foods at the bottom of the list have a higher carbohydrate content. In the third column, we divide the amount of calories by the protein content to get an index number. The lower the index number, the less calories and the more protein we get from that food. One hundred grams of the food is the equivalent to approximately one-fourth pound of food, or, for those with a food scale, a 3.5 ounce weight measurement. The percentage of protein is also the amount of grams of protein you will get from 100 grams of that particular food.

As you can see from the table, a heavy reliance on a typical American diet with anti-meat tendencies such as rice, French fries, pasta (noodles) bread, potatoes, oatmeal, etc., results in protein deficiency in the body.

To get 68 grams of protein (requirement for a 150-pound person), you could eat five eggs and you would be consuming only 790 calories. You will feel full too! If you didn't feel full, you still could have 710 calories to eat to reach the daily target of 1,500!

To get the same amount of protein from vegetable protein, you would need to eat 2.6 pounds of baked beans (a whopping 1,396 calories) or eat six pounds of rice (an astounding 2,700 calories!). This scenario reminds us of the breakfast cereal commercial where they bring in 35 bowls of cereal to the scared man in his pajamas to show how much cereal he would have to eat to get the same amount of fiber in one bowl of the cereal being promoted. Can you imagine having to eat six pounds of rice or 2.6 pounds of beans? Calorie disaster aside, it just won't work. It would be fattening, frustrating, and well, 2.6 pounds of beans? Scary.

You can change your diet to take in less than 1,200 calories per day, but if your calorie requirement is 2,500 calories per day, then you will create a caloric deficit in the amount of 1,300 calories per day. Due to the calorie deficit, your body will burn your existing body fat supply to get the energy from those calories. To get 1,300 calories worth of energy, it will require one-third pound of fat to be burned per day (or three pounds in 10 days, or nine pounds in a month).

To achieve a 1,200-calorie diet, for the purpose of weight loss, eat only the high-protein low-calorie foods from the previous table with an index of below 20. You will find that high-protein foods are "appetite suppressants." Because if you eat food supplying your protein requirement you will not be hungry anymore for the rest of the day, even if you did not get your calorie requirement. *Let your body be your guide.* Pay attention to your calorie and protein intake, but most importantly, listen to and understand your body's signals. It knows what it needs or, more importantly what it doesn't need, better than anyone.

The Big Secret: How to Stop Hunger and Cravings

Why do those hunger pangs hit? Why are you left unsatisfied and craving unhealthy and unfulfilling snacks that leave you feeling guilty or bloated? You really want the secret? You already know it! The big secret is that your body is hungry for protein! Your body does not want carbohydrates, but everyone seems to be turning to high-carbohydrate, high-calorie or low-fat foods. Then they remain hungry or become hungry again shortly after eating and make the mistake of eating more carbohydrates. Your body still feels hungry because it's protein requirement have not been met, causing it to ask for more and more and more. Give the body a lot of protein and your hunger and cravings disappear for the day. Worth a try, right? Say goodbye to those cravings between breakfast and lunch, between lunch and dinner, and between dinner and bedtime. They were never your friend and you don't need them in your life anymore!

Here are a just a few examples of meal ideas (and helpful hints) that are high in protein and low in carbohydrates.

BREAKFAST

Food: Four eggs your style (scrambled, fried, over easy, boiled, etc.)
Protein: 24 grams
Calories: 300

While losing weight, stay away from deviled eggs. Mayonnaise is a fatty 300 calories per ounce!

FOOD	CALORIES PER 100 GRAMS	PROTEIN PERCENTAGE	INDEX
Cod fish	70	17	4.4
Tuna fish	217	27.7	7.8
Chicken	175	20	8.8
Lean ham	136	25	9.4
Whole egg	158	12	12.3
Lamb	230	18	12.
Cheddar cheese	393	24	16.4
Beef roast	300	18	16.7
Cottage cheese	367	19	19.3
Whole milk	69	3.5	19.7
Beans baked	117	5.7	20.5
Cooked old-fashioned oats (oatmeal)	62	2.8	22.1
Whole-wheat bread	262	9.5	27.6
Fresh corn	108	3.7	29.2
Almonds	640	18.6	34.4
Cooked corn meal	59	1.4	42.1
Cooked noodles	385	2.0	45.0
Cooked rice	100	2.2	45.5
French fried potatoes	160	2.3	57.0

LUNCH

Food: One-half pound turkey, chicken, ham, lean ground beef, lamb, fish (tuna or cod) with a green salad.

Protein: 52 grams

Calories: 500

Wild fish, lamb, or grass-fed ground beef meat is preferred, as it contains more omega-3s than their alternates.

Be VERY careful with salad dressing, one ounce or 30 grams of oil can contain more than 300 calories.

Lemon juice and salt make a great salad dressing with no calories.

DINNER

Food: In the evening, eat those "negative calorie," non-starch vegetables all you want: broccoli, cabbage, carrots, mushrooms, peppers, squash, etc.

A beer or glass of wine, preferably red, is okay too.

If you are a 167-pound person, this daily menu gives you all of the protein you need to feel energized and you still will be under the 1,200 calorie mark, so you will rapidly lose weight.

When your weight returns to a normal, healthy range for your body type, you can start including some dark breads, fries or pastas, but keep your calorie intake to no more than your daily calorie requirement, or the weight will start to creep back up. After returning to a healthy weight, your food still should be predominantly high in protein and low in calories and carbohydrates.

When Dr. Schep was losing weight, he allowed himself one free day per week (like a holiday). On that day he could eat anything he wanted: chocolate cake, fries, pizza. It usually was on Saturdays. Beer and pizza after the football game or having a barbecue, etc. This did not affect his weight loss. However, he did find that because he had adequate protein intake for the six days preceding the free day, he could not eat that much anyway! His appetite was satisfied and his body was used to needing less gas to fill the tank.

Objections to Animal Protein

When we encourage people to eat animal protein, there usually are two immediate objections: The offended party is a vegetarian or a vegan; or those who insist increasing animal protein consumption would increase their cholesterol to dangerous levels. Let's address these concerns one by one.

We have been noticing a trend in the United States where some people (schoolteachers, the media, etc.) are teaching children and the public that eating animal protein is wrong because animals have to be killed. As a result, we are seeing an increasing number of people, especially women, with poor skin, weakened muscles, depression, bloated mid-sections, lethargy and many more symptoms that attack the rest of the body. These symptoms are occurring because of insufficient protein consumption on a daily basis. The skin is made from protein and it replaces itself every month. If you have insufficient protein intake, your skin is not able to fully regenerate, leaving you with discoloration, dryness, redness, itchi-

Please do note that while 1,200 calories is a safe and manageable daily calorie intake level, we don't recommend consuming less than that amount daily. If you feel that a daily calorie intake of less than 1,200 calories would benefit you, please discuss it with your doctor.

ness, blemishes, etc.

The cosmetic industry is making billions by engineering peptides in creams and lotions in order to try and get the protein back into the skin because women are not eating animal protein. By selling peptides for $30 or $40 dollars per one or two grams of content in a four-ounce jar, they are, in essence, selling you a steak for $5,000 that you can't even eat. Currently, the top selling anti-aging creams are selling for as much as $120 per bottle.

The peptides contained in these creams are incomplete forms of protein, and must get through the skin and into the body to have any cosmetic effect on your skin. You might be wondering why we are comparing fancy anti-aging peptide creams to steak? It is because by EATING a little steak and other animal proteins, your skin has the natural ability to regenerate and rectify underlying problems like redness, irritation, minor blemishes, etc., all on its own. And you have the enjoyment of a nice meal to boot.

This vegetarian attitude arose predominantly in the Orient, such as India. The vegetarian philosophy considers it wrong to kill animals and they must be left to live out their lives in peace, just as we do. At first glance, this philosophy seems to be in harmony with nature, but this is actually incorrect. Since the beginning of time on Earth, there has been a natural hierarchy of evolution with the carnivores being on the top of the food chain. The natural order of things, from that time forward, has looked something like this:

Grass-eating or herbivorous animals (livestock) were created to eat grass and other plant life.

That ingested plant life provides the necessary nutrients to help the herbivorous animals grow.

The nutrients then ferment in the animal's stomach and the bacteria uses it to make protein.

The protein provides us with nutrient-rich meat (not to mention, saving humans the trouble of eating a wheelbarrow full of grass or hay each day in order to survive).

One of the main purposes of animals is to assist in the circle of plant and human life. If all humans did not eat meat, the world would not need herbivorous animals around. This process is referred to as the food chain.

The big difference between the philosophy of Easterners and Westerners is that some Easterners think that if you withdraw from life and try and live as quiet an existence as possible, sitting in a cave and meditating all day, hardly eating and interacting with your surroundings, you will grow and evolve.

We don't see it quite that way. We Westerners believe that the more you live, the more active you are and the more you experience, the more you will learn and evolve. This is why the West has gotten so far ahead of the East in terms of prosperity and achievement.

We hope we have helped you understand the harm you can cause to your body, your health and your joints by not consuming sufficient high-quality proteins in your diet.

Most importantly, lack of quality protein makes your body unable to suppress your appetite. If you eat carbohydrates when you get hungry, it does not suppress your appetite; your blood sugar is always high; you just get fatter and fatter; your joints deteriorate;

and you could die earlier by suffering from arthritis, diabetes, heart disease and cancer. We know that reintroducing meat into your diet may be hard, but dying from heart disease and cancer due to lack of animal protein in your diet is even harder.

The Hard Truth About Animals and Vegetarians

If you still believe that the eating of animal protein is inhumane and that a strictly vegetarian diet should be followed in order to save the lives of innocent animals, the information in this section is going to shock you. Studies have shown that more animals are killed each year by the effects of following a vegetarian diet than by following a diet that includes meats. This following example may be extreme, but it perfectly illustrates the point. Dr. Schep became aware of the following situation because he was sitting on the Board of the Los Angeles Audubon Society as Executive Past President.

In the spring of 2006, there were 12,000 tricolored blackbirds in the San Jacinto Wildlife Preserve of Southern California. Populations of this species have significantly declined during the last century because of wetland destruction. Conservationists were puzzled because the birds were not nesting at the preserve like they normally had done over the past many years. However, in June, a tip came in that the birds had moved to a 13-acre wheat field approximately three miles away and had formed a nesting colony with about 6,000 chicks, representing about half the previous year's total population.

The farmer was determined to harvest the wheat and would destroy all the nests and kill all the chicks because they were interfering with his livelihood — the harvesting of his crop. Fortunately, the Audubon Society intervened on the birds' behalf and paid the farmer for his wheat crop. The farmer then ceased harvesting, therefore stopping the destruction of thousands of birds. If this had not happened, the hardcore and misdirected vegetarians eating the bread harvested from this acreage would have killed 6,000 birds — half the population of the species!

The lesson in this story is that, today, in America, wildlife are being driven out of their native environments due to overpopulation and new construction that is eating up the available fields, plains and forests that animals call their home. This development drives the animals into more populated areas and areas that closely resemble their homes — namely farms. There are several dangers for animals on farms. For example: Electric fences to keep out (or in) animals can cause serious injuries and burns that can get infected, and even cause death by shock to smaller animals. Pesticides used on the crops cause disease and death in the animals who are just looking for a meal. Harvesting equipment can run over and severely wound or kill animals, especially the smaller ones like bunnies, voles and mice. Our point is not that vegetarians are responsible for the death of these animals, but that we all should be aware of the processes from which our animal-free crops come and, in fact, the processes do cause harm to not only animals but the environment where the animals need to survive.

Take into consideration a meat eater. Eating beef grown on a 13-acre pasture instead of a wheat field would result in the death of only one or two animals, and these certainly are not endangered animal species.

Also, almost every part of the animal (beef) is used to make food, clothing, shoes and more. This scenario more closely resembles the natural, healthy way that our forefathers ate: Hunt, kill, eat and use the entire animal.

Although this is an extreme example and may be difficult for vegetarians to read. The fact is — birds, rabbits, moles and field mice regard a wheat field the same as they do a wild prairie and will make their homes there. Their homes and the animals themselves are destroyed when the wheat is harvested. As a vegetarian, all animals, even field mice, should get the same respect and generate the same outcry for humanity — even if they are not cute and cuddly.

The Least Harm Principle suggests that humans should eat beef, lamb and dairy, not a vegan diet. (S.L. Davis, Department of Animal Sciences, Oregon State University, Corvallis, OR 97331, writing for the Proceedings of the Third Congress of the European Society for Agricultural and Food Ethics, 2001, pp 449-450."). More information on the Least Harm Principal can be found at *http://www.freerepublic.com/focus/news/972951/posts.*

The Cholesterol Myth
The second concern to address is the idea that eating animal protein such as beef and eggs, will overload your body with cholesterol and eventually kill you. This is a myth also, and is promoted by those that sell cholesterol medications.

If you hatch an egg, the chick will be born in perfect health and will not be gasping and staggering around with hardened arteries. That sounds funny, but really think about it: That egg has all the nutrition in it to produce a perfect, healthy chick and that is why we say an egg is a perfect food. That chick is perfectly capable of surviving without supplemental food or milk from day one if it is the offspring of a bird species, such as game birds, that produce precocious young.

Agriculture kills more animals than cattle farming.

This is how the cholesterol myth started. Researchers in the early part of the last century wanted to find out why humans got hardened arteries or atherosclerosis. The researchers took guinea pigs and fed them a diet of fatty foods until the animals got atherosclerosis. The researchers then analyzed the food and found it had a high cholesterol content. What they failed to consider was the fact that there were numerous other factors in this diet that would cause atherosclerosis. The fatty foods had no vitamin C, no vitamin E, no omega-3 fatty acids, and no minerals such as copper — all of which would prevent inflammation in the veins and arteries by making and protecting protein such as elastin and collagen that the arteries themselves consist of. In a very negligent way, the scientists (in a very unscientific way), picked the cholesterol as the culprit; something, which has nothing to do with the actual inflammation of the arteries. From this study, the researchers created the theory of "good cholesterol" and "bad cholesterol" — *HDL and LDL.* The great cholesterol myth was then born. Pharmaceutical companies are perpetuating this myth in order to make billions of dollars annually from "statin" drugs, which actually interfere with the metabolism of your body and aggravate heart disease.

In spite of this information, the fact is available and clear for everybody to see:

People with a low or normal cholesterol content have just as much heart disease as people with a high blood cholesterol content.

In greater detail, around 1963, researchers (as reported by Klevay[14] 1985) induced atherosclerosis in mice by feeding them a diet high in saturated fat. The diet consisted of 58 percent sugar, 28 percent lard and a salt mixture called USP XIII No.

Meat Versus No Meat

Regan the Vegan, mentioned in these Web sites (*http://www.webster.edu/~corbetre/philosophy/ animals/regan-text.htm*l and *http://www. thevegetariansite.com/ethics_regan.htm*) is against the use of animals for food and he appears to be totally unaware of the fact that a cattle pasture kills less animals and gives more animals and birds a home than a cornfield or a wheatfield. He is therefore in logical conflict.

S.L Davis is presently online at *http://www. freerepublic.com/focus/news/972951/posts*. In the Davis versus Regan the Vegan argument, we side with Davis. A cornfield, if it replaces a pasture or a wildlife area, is a wasteland for animals. Even crows are shot by farmers if they dare venture on a cornfield. Plus, in this book we show how ruinous corn-based syrup is to our health. A cattle pasture, however, has myriad animals in it, especially if it has trees to provide shade for the cows and streams. A pasture is very similar to a savanna, a treeless plain that has been around for millions of years. IN Africa, buffalo, zebra and wildebeest roam in the savannas and all kinds of birds, rodents and other mammals live there as well. It is much more natural than a cornfield. The cornfield also is less productive than a pasture because only the ears are harvested. It lies fallow and unproductive for most of the year and no animal will go near it. Cattle eat in a pasture, the entire grass, not just the grain. Also, as noted above, any creatures that do inhabit an agricultural field will be disrupted or killed, or will have to leave when the field is harvested and plowed under. The pasture remains home for animals the entire year because it supplies food in the form of roots, leaves, bulbs nuts and seeds.

2 Salt Mixture.

This mineral mix does not supply the essential minerals: manganese, zinc, copper, iodine, chromium and selenium. The calcium level is low. MP recommends the use of supplement U.S.P. XIII, No. 2 Mineral Mix in conjunction with this formulation for long-term growth and development of the rat.

Deaths due to atrial thrombosis began to occur after nine weeks on the diet and after 18 weeks only a few mice were still alive. The arteries of the mice were analyzed and found to be loaded with cholesterol. So the researchers proposed we stay away from saturated fat and cholesterol. That means meat, milk and eggs, the very things our bodies need to fight disease, stay lean and inflammation free!

However, then came Doctor L.M. Klevay[14], 1985, animal nutritionist for the United States Department of Agriculture (USDA). He noticed that the diet was deficient in copper, so he fed the mice that same sugar, lard and salt diet, but added copper to their drinking water. He reported that most of the mice that received the sugar lard and salt diet, **with** added copper in their drinking water, were still alive after 18 weeks. He proved that animal fats and lard DID NOT cause heart disease by promoting the cholesterol in the body, but that the thrombosis was caused by a deficiency of copper in the diet. Copper promotes the protecting copper-containing enzyme, superoxide dismutase (SOD) — The enzyme that protects the arteries against free radicals and inflammation by causing the destructive MMPs to back off. Copper also promotes the formation of healthy elastin protein, assuming, of course, that you eat a good-quality protein diet with lysine (the essential amino acid we talked about earlier). The enzyme that makes the elastin tissue in healthy arteries is called *lysyl oxidase*, and it is a copper-containing enzyme.

We now know that omega-3 fatty acids also prevent inflammation in the arteries, and that saturated fats do not contain omega-3 fatty acids. Therefore, the cholesterol theory is pseudoscience (speculation based upon an improper interpretation of the results of experiments), or just a plain lousy experiment with the wrong salt and mineral mix.

One precaution, however. Farmers sometimes give their animals antibiotics, which lessens the amount of bacteria in the gut and causes the animals to grow faster and bigger and produce more meat. It's the same reason they give chickens antibiotics. Some farmers, however, fear the bacteria will become resistant to antibiotics and feed the chickens arsenic instead to achieve the same purpose. The problem with arsenic is that unless you take a sufficient amount of vitamin C (2,000 milligrams), which detoxifies the body, the arsenic accumulates in your body and is a carcinogen. Consumer Union analyzed chicken meat and found arsenic in all chicken, except that from organically produced chicken or Foster Farms chicken, *http://www.fosterfarms.com*. When buying chicken, go for organic whenever possible and ensure you are getting enough vitamin C. You can view the report at: *http://www.consumerreports.org/cro/food/food-safety/animal-feed-and-food/animal-feed-and-the-food-supply-105/chicken-arsenic-and-antibiotics/*.

You will note in the Web site that the Food and Drug Administration (FDA) allows 500 micrograms per kilogram of arsenic in chickens but the Environmental Protection Agency (EPA) does not. Go figure.

Body Repair and Food Digestion
"Macroautophagy" is a major repair process for membranes and cell structures damaged by reactive oxygen species (ROS), otherwise known as free radicals (Bergamini[57]). Dur-

U.S.P. XIII No. 2 Salt Mixture

INGREDIENT	AMOUNT
Calcium Biphosphate	13.58%
Calcium Lactate	32.69%
Ferric Citrate (16-17% Fe)	2.96%
Magnesium Sulfate	13.70%
Potassium Phosphate Dibasic	23.99%
Sodium Biphosphate	8.73%
Sodium Chloride	4.35%

Reference: United States Pharmacopeia (USP) XIII, 1945, 721. MP Biomedical catalog, *http://www.mpbio.com/product_info.php?open=products&cPath=1_16_130&selecttab=&family_key=02902845*

ing this process, the damaged cell structure is surrounded by pieces of cell membrane and its molecular components are recycled. This process is reduced after eating because insulin and amino acids rise, meaning that cellular repair likely only occurs during fasting (Mortimore G. E.[58]). By reducing insulin levels, CRON sets the stage for more cellular repair (Bergamini E. et al 2003; Droge W. 2004).

Therefore, eating excess carbohydrates causes the body to produce more insulin, slowing the cellular repair process. This holds for both tissue and joints. Also, what follows from this is that we should eat a few meals a day (two to three), so that when we don't eat, the body can rebuild itself. Eat dinner early and then nothing till breakfast. You cannot clean the ash out of a furnace while it is burning!

The Occupational Safety and Health Agency (OSHA) allows only 10 micrograms of arsenic per cubic meter in the workplace air for eight hours of exposure. That's 143 micrograms inhaled. If you allowed your employees to bring and eat chicken to the workplace with the FDA allowable amount of arsenic in it, namely 250 micrograms per pound, you could be severely fined by OSHA if they followed the law to the letter.

THE DIET SUMMARY

There is a lot of information in this chapter, but remember how easy it is to shrink your problem areas and live a healthier, more energetic, satisfied life without succumbing to cravings and feeling guilty.

The formula is easy: Reduce the carbohydrates, increase the protein and stay between 1,200 and 1,500 calories per day (for weight loss). And most important of all — Get rid of that white sugar. There are a lot of poisons being given to the hazardous waste department that are less toxic than white sugar.

Please believe that if we can do it, you can do it. Have faith in yourself and challenge yourself to find new, delicious, creative ways to cook and eat. You can do this and, in doing so, you will feel incredible! Your body will move better, feel better, you will sleep better, and your mind will be at ease because you won't be thinking about food all the time. Make this change and you will never regret it.

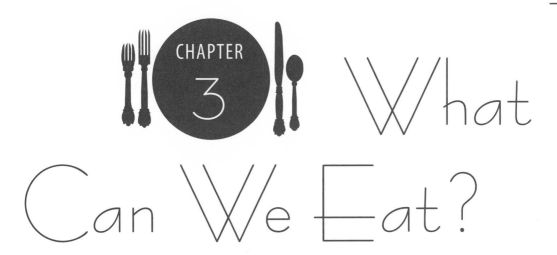

CHAPTER 3 What Can We Eat?

There are no perfect foods (other than maybe eggs). Every food is lacking in some nutrient or other. This means that a well-balanced variety is key. Sadly, some people choose a small limited variety of food and stick to it, eating the same six or seven foods, day after day, never daring to eat anything different for the rest of their lives. It is clear then that these persons will be much more likely to have nutritional deficiencies.

In this chapter, we will address the major diseases of the industrialized world, namely heart disease, cancer, osteoporosis, arthritis, obesity, aging, diabetes and infectious diseases. We will show how these diseases are a result of foods that have been altered and chemically engineered by the food companies so that they are no longer in the form intended by nature.

The best way to eliminate these diseases and prevent them from happening is to change our diet to include the proper vitamins, minerals and nutrients. There are many nutrients lacking in the present day American diet, but our focus is on the most problematic, which are the lack of copper and omega-3 fatty acids. The next most important nutrients that we need to start reincorporating into our diets are vitamin C, anti-oxidants, and fiber.

We have shown without a doubt that copper is lacking in our diets and that this lack is unquestionably the most serious factor in heart disease. It also has been shown that copper deficiency is probably the most unknown and next greatest factor in cancer. What is important to know, but hasn't been widespread until now, is that copper and anti-oxidants both have the same function in the cell, namely removal of free radicals that disrupt the cell function (i.e. cancer and heart disease, two of our nation's top killers).

Knowing this information, we should be maintaining a proper diet rich in nutrients so that we can stave off these serious diseases and stay strong and healthy. In addition to copper, protein, vitamins, anti-oxidants and essential amino acids are also critical in building and maintaining the proper dietary balance. What our bodies don't need, however, are carbohydrates and sugar! Unfortunately, the average American daily diet contains approximately 60 to 70 percent carbohydrates.

WELL-BALANCED VARIETY IS KEY

The problem we face is that the snack and prepackaged food industry, "Big Food," tries to shove sugar and carbohydrates down our throats because they make billions of dollars a year off the American public. We are busy and tired, and their commercials play on our yearning for fast, efficient meals and snacks that "the whole family will love." They even trick us by using additives (most often chemical-based) to make the foods smell more like fresh, natural food. It's also what they do to dog food!

At this point you probably are wondering what foods you can eat. Not to worry, there are an abundance of fresh, natural, easy-to-prepare foods readily available that contain everything nature intended your body to have without artificial fillers.

The No.1 rule — eat unprocessed foods. Unprocessed foods are those that clearly have not been tampered with (i.e. prepackaged foods, with some exceptions like kombu and some nuts). In Chapter 4, Why Raw Is Better, we will give you a whole list of unprocessed foods that are easy to find at the store and easy to prepare, but here are a few great examples of low-carbohydrate, high-protein meals. The meals with a star (★) are also gluten free!

Did you know that Eskimos didn't eat carbohydrates? All that was available to arctic Eskimos was animal protein and fat (before food stamps were invented). The Eskimo's bodies utilized the protein to make all the glucose (in the liver) that their brains needed. Even better, their food was loaded with omega-3, which means that they did not suffer from diseases such as heart disease, arthritis, cancer and hypertension. The omega-3 also made their skin smooth, supple and radiant, even in the harshest weather conditions.

Breakfast

★2 eggs scrambled with 1 ounce grated cheese and 2 slices turkey bacon or lean★ turkey breast.

★5-egg omelet with sliced bell peppers and onions.

★One cup cottage cheese with sliced peaches or other fresh or frozen fruits.

★3 hard-boiled eggs with 2 slices of fruit.

3 slices rye toast with 1 tablespoon organic peanut butter on each.

Lunch

Salad rolls (lettuce, avocado, sliced carrots and other fresh veggies wrapped in Romaine lettuce leaves).

★4 slices lean meat filled with cream cheese or hummus.

★Tossed salad with grilled chicken breast, fresh tomatoes and cucumbers, or other veggies of choice.

★Grilled chicken breast with 1 ounce melted mozzarella cheese and side salad.

Burrito made with pinto beans, melted cheese and wrapped in a corn or low carbohydrate tortilla.

Dinner

10-ounce grilled salmon steak with asparagus and a glass of red wine or fresh iced tea.

8-ounce beef steak with steamed fresh vegetables.

10-ounce lemon pepper chicken breast with steamed, mashed cauliflower (faux mashed potatoes).

8-ounce seasoned pork chop with 1 cup quinoa.

1 cup whole-wheat or low-carbohydrate spaghetti with ½ cup organic spaghetti sauce and broccoli bits.

As you can see from some of the examples, the foods our bodies crave are readily available at our local stores, cost less (on average) than the prepackaged unhealthy foods we are eating now, and taste so much better than what we are grabbing through the drive through. Most all of the meals listed above are easily prepared in advance or only take about 30 minutes to bake, broil or grill. We like to make a few of these meals on Saturday or Sunday and package them into individual servings, then we don't have to think about meal planning, especially what to eat for breakfast (that seems to be the most challenging) for the rest of the week.

A great thing about restaurants is that they have an abundance of unprocessed and fresh food available to order. However, you do have to be cautious about how the food is prepared at restaurants. If things are boiled in tap water (fluoride), cooked in an aluminum pot or fried in aluminum pans (aluminum), the health of the food is not as high as if it was prepared using stainless steel. Sometimes, you can't be sure what is going on in the kitchen, but it is more than okay to specify to the waiter that you want the food prepared lightly, without butters and heavy sauces. You can specify the cooking method too. For instance, ask for your meat broiled instead of baked, or grilled instead of boiled. Most restaurants aim to please, so they will make every effort to prepare your food in the way you ask them to. That's what keeps you coming back to their restaurant!

COPPER IN THE DIET

Copper is one of the best minerals for your body. It creates elastin tissue (what your heart and arteries are made of), helps prevent arterial plaque, is a natural beta blocker and it prevents cancer by making an SOD enzyme that destroys superoxide radicals. When choosing foods and vitamins, copper usually isn't on the top of our "wish list," but it should be. It is very important to incorporate foods that are naturally high in copper into our diets to help maintain a healthy heart.

To naturally incorporate copper in your daily diet, try adding these foods (the foods at the top of the list have the highest copper content):

Shellfish, especially oysters
Liver
Blackstrap molasses
Dark chocolate
Sunflower seeds
Sesame seeds
Sunflower seeds
Pumpkin seeds
Nuts (especially cashews and then almonds)

OMEGA-3 AND OMEGA-9

To begin adding Omega-3s back into your diet, try:

Wild fish (such as salmon and sardines)
Canola oil
Chia seeds
Hempseed oil
Flaxseed oil
Olive oil (omega-9)
Safflower oil (omega-9)

VITAMIN C

Vitamin C is essential for your immune system, it is rich in anti-oxidants that fight free radicals and it fortifies many functions of the body. Humans are one of the few species that cannot make their own internal vitamin C supply, so it is especially important for us to include it in our diets. Add the following foods into your diet to boost your vitamin C intake:

Oranges
Grapefruit
Watermelons
Acerola powder
Red, yellow and orange bell peppers
Broccoli
Tomatoes
Papaya
Mango
Peas
Cauliflower
Watercress
Spinach

ANTI-OXIDANTS

Anti-oxidants fight free radicals and diseases and fortify our immune systems. Luckily, anti-oxidants are found in these delicious, carotene-rich (vitamin A) foods:

Carrots
Sweet potatoes
Pumpkins
Squashes (especially winter squash)
Beets
Blueberries
Goji berries
Strawberries
Cherries
Dark chocolate
Turmeric
Cloves (Turmeric and cloves have the highest amounts of anti-oxidants)

Cruciferous vegetables that contain anti-oxidants as well as sulforaphanes, which are agents that encourage our bodies to pro-

duce anti-oxidants, include:

Cabbage, especially red cabbage
Broccoli
Brussels sprouts
Watercress
Mustard greens
Collard greens
Turnips
Radishes
Kohlrabi
Sauerkraut (the best)

PROTEIN

Easy to digest and complete sources of protein, include:

Fish
Beef
Pork
Eggs
Chicken
Turkey

We recommend cooking your protein by methods other than frying, barbecuing or grilling if possible. Carnosine, the anti-aging, anti-glycating and anti-cancer compound found in protein, can be destroyed during the frying process.

Vegetarian Protein

As an alternate to meat, a combination of healthy grains, vegetables and beans can supply you with complete protein. Although, if you choose to get your protein requirement solely from grains, beans and nuts, this may cause your calorie intake to become higher than is healthy or practical for your waistline.

To make sure your vegetarian diet contains enough protein, ensure your daily diet includes some of the following protein sources:

Eggs (the best source of protein)

Nuts

Broccoli

Lentils

Brown rice

Bulgur

Beans

PROBIOTICS

The Food and Agricultural Organization (FAO) of the United Nations and the World Health Organization (WHO), define probiotics as "live microorganisms, which when administered in adequate amounts, confer a beneficial health effect on the host." In laymen's terms, probiotics are live, healthy bacteria that help our bodies when consumed. Probiotics are mainly used to help regulate the digestive system and keep your colon and intestines healthy and functioning regularly.

Yogurt is the best source for probiotics although, if you are brave, you could try some fermented milk, which is commonly used in European cultures. When buying yogurt, make sure the label mentions "probiotics" or "live cultures." Unpasteurized sauerkraut and mild kimchi are also sources of probiotics.

FIBER

Fiber is important not only for sustaining the bowel and regulating your digestive system, but for increasing strength and energy as well. Whole oats supply fiber and complex carbohydrates. It is unique in the fact that oats can increase testosterone levels by blocking sex hormone-binding globulin, thereby providing strength and energy. To stay regular and increase your energy, include these sources of fiber in your diet:

Whole bran flakes (can supply 25 grams of fiber per cup)

Whole (not pearl) barley (whole barley can supply up to 14 grams of fiber per cup and contains vitamin E)

Rice bran (has a high anti-oxidant value)

Chia seeds (contain the most fiber at 38 grams fiber per 3.5 ounces of seeds!)

Beans

Broccoli

Spinach

Kale

Bok choy

Cruciferous vegetables

FOOD SUBSTITUTIONS

Sometimes the hardest part of following a new diet or plan is knowing that we need to change the way we eat, but not knowing how to do it. This can leave us frustrated, which can ultimately lead to failure. Here is a handy list of substitutions for common grocery or convenience items that will help you stay on track and make the supermarket a less stressful experience.

FOOD	RECOMMENDED SUBSTITUTION(S)
White sugar	Blackstrap molasses (highest mineral content); Splenda; maple syrup; Stevia
White rice	Brown rice (high in minerals and vitamin B)
White flour	Whole-wheat flour (high in minerals and vitamin B; rice flour
White bread	Whole-wheat bread
Beef (corn fed)	Organic, grass-fed beef (high in omega-3)
Black/green tea	Rooibos (Red Bush) tea (powerful anti-oxidants, caffeine free) Also known as African red tea (Starbucks has it!)
Potato chips/snack crackers	Nuts: brazil, cashew, almond, goji (contains copper and selenium); Chia seeds; sugar snap peas (fruits and veggies provide anti-oxidants); dried, unsweetened fruit; fresh fruits and vegetables; whole-wheat crackers
French fries	Fresh or steamed vegetables; baked potato (with olive oil and vegetables); side salad; broth-based soup; brown rice
White wine	Red wine (anti-oxidants)
Salad dressing	Lemon juice (low calorie) and olive oil or safflower oil (omega-9); red wine vinegar (low calorie)
Corn oil/sunflower oil	Canola oil (omega-3) Hempseed oil (omega-3)
Milk chocolate	Dark chocolate — 60 percent or higher chocolate content (copper, minerals, anti-oxidants)
Doughnuts	Fresh fruit; whole-grain bread with peanut butter

FOOD	RECOMMENDED SUBSTITUTION(S)
Fatty dips	Hummus; bean dips
Candy	Raisins; nuts; dates (minerals, fiber, anti-oxidants)
Regular pizza	Use whole-wheat crust with more vegetables, olives, pineapple, more tomato, less processed meats (less calories, more minerals and anti-oxidants)
White pasta	Whole-wheat pasta
Fried meats	Boiled, baked or stewed meats (watch the temperature!)
Soda	Water; lemonade; sugar-free fruit juice; sparkling water; almond milk; tea; fresh-made orange juice (store-bought is pasteurized)
Juice with added sugar	Zero sugar added juice
Processed cheese slices	Block cheese
Energy drinks	Added vitamins and minerals
Side salad	Cole slaw
Onion rings	Steamed vegetables
White flour tortillas	Corn tortillas
Cream-based soups	Broth-based soups
Store-bought trail mix with candy pieces	Homemade trail mix with unprocessed nuts, dried fruits and no candy pieces

CHAPTER 4 Why Raw is Better

Raw foods such as carrots, celery, cherry tomatoes, broccoli, cauliflower, apples, grapes, melons, and oranges are some our favorite snacks. These snacks are low-fat, low-calorie, guilt-free and delicious. They also help fight breast cancer, prostate cancer, and help protect your skin from harmful UV rays from the inside out! We'll show you how to snack your way into a lean, clean healthy machine! Fruits and vegetables are not your only raw food options.

Raw foods don't always have to be eaten raw You can cook them, dress them and make delicious meals out of them. However, it is important to know that the heating of food is not beneficial and nutrients and minerals in the food actually can be harmed by the cooking process. In this chapter we will teach you how to cook and prepare food in a way that minimizes the loss of all the healthy benefits contained in the raw product. Although it is not practical for most people to go on a raw food diet, it is emphasized that we must include some raw food in our diets at least once a day. Oysters, pickled herring (don't knock it 'till you try it!), sashimi, and jerky can be included.

Eating raw food means eating uncooked and unprocessed foods. The raw food purists state that enzymes in food start to degrade at temperatures as low as 102 F and are completely degraded at 126 F. So, true raw food is food that has not been heated in any way, including microwaving. The process of exposing food to ionizing radiation to destroy such things as bacteria, insects, and viruses — irradiation — is also used to delay ripening in foods and increase food hydration. It is considered unhealthy because, if the radiation can disrupt the cells of microbes, it can also alter the nutrients in the food and produce harmful free radicals.

The Food and Drug Administration (FDA) requires irradiated food to have a symbol on the package, which is a green circle with two leaves and a dot in it. It is called the Radura symbol. The symbol is similar to the logo of the United States Environmental Protection Agency (EPA). Fruit and vegetables that are not packaged must have the symbol displayed when it is ready for sale by stores or markets.

Raw foods include dried foods, pickled foods, refrigerated foods, sprouted seeds, frozen foods and fermented foods. There are raw vegans that exclude all animal products and raw vegetarians that will drink raw milk and eat raw cheese. There are even raw food eaters that avoid grains and beans because of digestibility, toxin issues, and the fact that these foods are Neolithic domesticated foods. The Neolithic period is when humans started using agriculture to domesticate and process wild foods. It is claimed that wild einkorn wheat, as opposed to domesticated wheat, has gliadin in it and it is not as toxic (compared to modern wheat) to people with celiac disease.

Heat occurs when a molecule takes up energy then starts to move faster. The faster it moves, the higher temperature it creates. If we heat water, the water molecules start moving faster and faster, colliding with each other more frequently. The speed of movement is called "temperature." The higher the speed, the higher the temperature. If we heat the water high enough, then these molecules start moving so fast that they literally shoot up through the surface of the water into the air above. This is called steam, and we say the water is boiling.

History of Cooking

Archeologists found the first human-like remains over two million years ago. Those archeologists state that there are signs that humans started cooking their food as many as 250,000 years ago. Before then, humans and animals alike ate only raw foods, namely raw fruits, vegetables, grains and meats. Today, wild animals continue to exist on a raw food diet while humans exist almost solely on cooked or processed foods. Wild animals do not have raging obesity, heart disease, diabetes and cancer rates, but the rates of those diseases in humans, especially Americans, is astronomical.

It is without question that raw foods are natural and healthy. We are seeing more and more movements promoting diets including only raw foods. These diets have a huge following and are even followed or endorsed by many celebrities, including Demi Moore, Uma Thurman, Jason Mraz, Carol Alt and Alicia Silverstone.

When solid molecules are heated, they start shaking and vibrating. If the shaking gets violent enough the molecules can break apart. It is like driving a car with an axle or wheels that are out of balance. The faster the car is driven the more it shakes. If you drive the car fast enough, eventually the car will fall apart. Likewise, heating food causes the molecules to shake and vibrate, distorting them and eventually breaking them apart.

It is without question that raw foods are the absolute best foods for you and that cooking them can greatly reduce their benefits. The reason: Heat destroys the molecular structure of food and it breaks down the molecules by either fragmenting, distorting and bending, or by causing the molecules to combine with each other. This also means without question that the higher the temperature the more the food is altered or destroyed.

Specifically, heat can destroy enzymes, vitamin C and anti-oxidants. It also converts good fats (CIS) into bad trans fats, breaks molecules into free radicals and generates cancerous "heterocyclic aromatic amines," which is the name given to char-forming chemicals in meat if it is cooked in high heat, such as flame cooking.

Consider the example of a kiln that makes the finest bricks for building houses. All the bricks are perfect and stack neatly in tidy piles. The bricklayer easily is able to take the bricks and make perfect straight walls that are strong. The next step is to transport the bricks to the building site in such a way that they maintain their shape and form. Now we have a truck driver who comes and loads the bricks in the back of his truck. Being under pressure, he flings the bricks in the back of his truck and some break. He then finds that he has to drive to some outlying area over a badly corrugated gravel road. Being in a hurry, the entire truck shakes and vibrates and by the time he gets to the building site, half the bricks are broken. He dumps the load right at the bricklayers feet. The bricklayer now has to

go through the pile of debris to find good bricks and it takes him twice as long to build the wall. Also, he did not notice some of the bricks had hidden cracks in them so the wall is now under strength and not capable of withstanding an earthquake or a heavy load. Even worse, the bricklayer now has to clean up the debris and load it into a dumpster and arrange to have it carted away.

Likewise, the body needs perfect building materials to build a healthy strong body. Nature supplies these perfect building blocks in our food. When we cook our food, a lot of the molecules are broken and shattered (like the bricklayer driving too fast over the gravel road). The more we cook our foods and the higher the temperature used, the more molecules that are rendered useless. The body now has to go through the process of sorting out all of the good molecules and disposing of all the broken unsuitable molecules. If some of the molecules are only slightly altered (like the cracked bricks) the body will still use them, but then you have a weakened and inferior body.

RAW FOOD FACTS

Raw food contains digestive enzymes such as amylases, proteases and lipases and these aid digestion.

Raw foods contain beneficial bacteria that suppress harmful bacteria in the gut.

Raw foods have higher nutrient values and anti-oxidants than cooked foods.

Cooked foods have toxins such as heterocyclic aromatic amines that promote cancer. Cooking oils that contain trans fats may also contain heterocyclic aromatic amines and cooking meat or any protein with sugar can glycate the protein making it unusable by the body.

Scientific research studies have shown that raw foods protect against such diseases as heart disease and cancer and decrease toxins in the colon.

Consuming raw vegetables and fruits lowers your risk for heart attacks, breast and colon cancer, diabetes and obesity.

Raw broccoli contains approximately 60 percent more vitamin C and 40 percent more vitamin A than cooked broccoli.

One clove of raw garlic contains almost as much antibacterial power as 100,000 units of penicillin.

Raw foods provide hydration and essential vitamins and nutrients that make our skin radiant and blemish free.

RAW FOODS AND YOUR THYROID

Certain raw foods contain goitrogens, a substance that interferes with the thyroid gland. Cooking destroys the enzymes that make the goitrogens, but bacteria in the stomach will always produce low levels of goitrogens naturally. If you have low thyroid (defined by a Thyroid-Stimulating Hormone or TSH test with above average rating) it might be wise to minimize these foods. You also can include a thyroid stimulator like kombu (contains iodine) and brazil nuts (contains selenium) in your diet to minimize or counter-act the effect of the goitrogen.

Following is a list of raw foods that have been identified as lightly goitrogenic. It is important to note that cooking these foods eliminates or reduces the goitrogen.

Soybeans (and soybean products such as tofu, soybean oil, soy flour, soy lecithin)

Pine nuts
Cassava
Peanuts
Millet
Strawberries
Pears
Peaches
Spinach
Bamboo shoots
Radishes
Horseradish
Sweet potatoes
Vegetables in the genus brassica
Bok choy
Broccoli
Broccolini (asparations)
Brussels sprouts
Cabbage
Canola
Cauliflower
Chinese cabbage
Choy sum
Collard greens
Kai-lan (Chinese broccoli)
Kale
Kohlrabi
Mizuna
Mustard greens
Rapeseed (yu choy)
Rapini
Rutabagas
Tatsoi
Turnips

MAKING THE MOST OF MEAT

Although we are not going to try and convince you to eat your meat raw, we are going to teach you that the way you cook your meats can make a dramatic difference to your health.

Researchers have found that one of the highest factors affecting the risk of cancer is the high temperature cooking of meat. They found that the highest quartile (25 percent) of fried meat and barbecued meat-eaters have a 400 percent greater risk of cancer than the lowest 25 percent of fried meat-eaters, as opposed to the same comparison between high sugar intake or low carotene intake where the risks vary from 100 to 200 percent. Those in the bottom 25 percent of carotene intake have a 200 percent higher risk than those that are in the 25 percent of highest carotene intake.

What does that mean in plain English? It means that if our diet consists of a high percentage of meats that are fried or cooked over an open flame, you are running a cancer risk 400 percent higher than people whose diet contains less than 25 percent of fried meat or meat cooked over an open flame. That is a HUGE percentage, and a HUGE risk to your health!

When meat is subjected to high temperatures, even enough to simply char it, the amino acids in the protein react with creatinine to form compounds called heterocyclic aromatic amines (HAA). The body then metabolizes these HAAs into compounds that bind to DNA, therefore mutating your cells and instigating your immune system to attack it and cause inflammation, which goes hand-in-hand with cancer.

Rashimi Sinha[59] of the National Cancer Institute reported that meat pan-fried at 212 F, the boiling point of water, had no HAA. Meat pan-fried at 420 F contained high amounts of HAA. This temperature easily can be and, often is, reached by grills and other open-flame cooking methods.

Because of the heath risk of frying meat over such high heats, it is scientifically and nutritionally recommended that you fry your meat in an electric skillet at a setting close to 212 F or lower. Also, try to avoid frying your meat at higher temperatures or barbecuing over an open flame. The maximum temperature that can be achieved by most skillets is 480 F. The best cooking levels for meat are rare or medium-rare and the consumption of barbecued meat should be kept to the absolute minimum. Barbecued

Allegations and the Real Truth About Certain Raw Foods

Statement: Raw beans have enzymes in them that inhibit the digestion of protein.

The Truth: Some beans may cause gas, which can inhibit digestion, and some people may have sensitivities to some raw beans such as fava beans. Cooking beans inactivates the beneficial enzymes, destroys the anti-oxidants (bad) and inactivates protease enzyme inhibitors (good). The protease enzyme is necessary to digest protein. (For example raw beans have an ORAC value of around 8,000, cooked beans have an ORAC value of 1,000 or less). So only cook beans enough to make them edible by destroying the inhibitor without destroying the anti-oxidants. (See kidney beans in Chapter 10.)

Statement: Raw alfalfa sprouts contain a toxin called canavanine. The plant makes this compound as an intermediate in the making of the amino acid, arginine.

The Truth: Research shows that when the sprouts turn green, this compound is reduced to a trace amount, eliminating any possible negative effects in the body. In addition, Dr. Rosenthal, of the University of Kentucky, found canavanine to protect against cancer.

Statement: Raw eggs contain avidin that inhibits biotin (vitamin B).

The Truth: You would have to eat as many as 24 raw eggs per sitting to inactivate or inhibit biotin.

Statement: Raw foods, particularly meat, milk and eggs, can contain harmful bacteria and/or toxins.

The Truth: Meats and organic milk products from grass-fed cattle contain much less bacteria and toxins than from cattle in crowded feedlots, and provide increased levels of vitamins, minerals, nutrients, amino acids and healthy enzymes.

meats are delicious, we know, but they drastically increase your risk of cancer and other diseases and it's not worth the 15 minutes of enjoyment for your taste buds.

Boiling is a great way to cook meat as you can control the temperature, the water source, the type of pot (stainless steel is preferable) and how well done the meat is. Boiled beef and turkey are great for making stews and chili, and boiled chicken can be seasoned and shredded for use on salads, in tacos or enchiladas. Borscht, a Russian stew, is especially healthy by combining boiled stewing meat with additional benefits of anti-oxidants and fiber from the beets.

The vegetarian's position is that no meat should be consumed whatsoever. We do understand their view, but the hard part of the vegetarian lifestyle is that they must get their protein only from grains, beans and nuts. This means that they are either protein deficient or they have to consume more calories than needed. To get adequate protein intake, they would have to take in hundreds, even thousands, of excess calories per day, which leads to obesity, glycation, heart disease and cancer. And, as we mentioned earlier, animals still get killed in the grain-harvesting process. The middle ground, the way nature intended us to eat, is a balanced combination of meat, grains, nuts, fruits and vegetables.

CRUCIFEROUS VEGETABLES

This family of plants is beneficial because they contain compounds called *glucosinolates*. Glucosinolates are indirectly responsible for their anti-cancer ability. Different members of the Brassica clan contain different forms and different amounts of glucosinolates, so it is important to incorporate different items

from the list and consume good amounts of these vegetables in your daily diet.

For example, if you make a salad or stir-fry with watercress for dinner tonight, make

Choosing a Cooking Skillet

When choosing an electric skillet, choose one with a stainless steel or ceramic cooking surface. Stay away from those made from plastics, such as Teflon or those with other non-stick coatings. We recommend purchasing an electric skillet with a temperature range starting as low as 186 F. Stainless steel skillets pots, pans and skillets are harder to clean if you are not used to them, but you can easily get those tough foods off by boiling plain water in the empty pan, then gently scrubbing the pan with stainless steel wool. If the residue is really stubborn, you can use powdered scouring cleaners, but make sure to thoroughly rinse the cleaner off with boiling hot water so no residue gets into your next meal. More often than not, boiling water in the pan and gently scrubbing will remove all tough food and residue.

a salad with kale and sliced radish for lunch tomorrow. The next day you could snack on raw chopped cauliflower and broccoli, or make faux mashed potatoes (see recipes in Chapter 10) as a side dish to fresh fish or chicken.

Cruciferous vegetables include the following vegetables:

Cabbage
Broccoli
Brussels sprouts
Cauliflower
Collards
Kale
Kohlrabi
Mibuna
Swede

Mustard

Rocket

Turnip

Wasabi

Watercress

Horseradish

Radish

Money plant (oh yes, there really is a money plant!)

How do the cancer-fighting properties of these plants work? When the plants are cut, ground or chewed, an enzyme in the plant called *myrosinase* is released. The myrosinase then reacts with the glucosinolates to form *isocyanates,* and indoles, both of which either prevent the formation of cancer-causing substances in the body or speed up the elimination of the cancer-causing substances from the body.

However, cooking destroys the myrosinase enzyme. Intestinal bacteria still can convert some glucosinolate to isocyanates, which happens in the digestive tract, but the transformation is greatly reduced. This is a prime example of how eating foods in their raw form promotes healthy bodies from the inside out.

Earlier we discussed cruciferous vegetables, which are not recommended for those that have a low thyroid output because they contain goitrogens. However, watercress, which is almost always eaten raw, is reported to have a good effect on the thyroid gland because of its high iodine content. Watercress, traditionally, has actually been used as a thyroid tonic. Try adding watercress to your salads or stir-fry, or try it alone as a snack. Sauerkraut (made from cabbage) also neutralizes the effects of the goitrogens. Both these vegetables make a delicious, disease-fighting snack or condiment. Not only do they taste great, they are crunchy enough to get the same satisfaction as munching chips or pretzels and much better for you!

BEEF JERKY

In the days of the pioneers when you were traveling great distances, you needed to be able to carry food with you that was easily portable and that gave you the protein and nutrients your body required to make the trip. That food was jerky! Jerky is a great snack that comes from preparing meat without any cooking whatsoever, thereby retaining the integrity and health benefits of the meat. While we cannot recommend jerky sold with the addition of sugar, sodium nitrite and other preservatives (no pioneer or wagon traveler would ever dream of ingesting those things), we are going to teach you how to make healthy, delicious, disease-fighting jerky.

Dr. Schep recommends the South African way of making jerky, which is used by the Voortrekkers in South Africa (his ancestors). The end product is called "Biltong." Any beef can be used to make jerky, and there is no advantage to using the more expensive cuts. See Chapter 10 for the Biltong recipe.

RAW MILK

Milk is another prime example of why raw is better. It is the perfect raw, animal protein. Although, there is one problem: The milk we consume today is not the same "food" that humans consumed for 10,000 years. Today's milk is intensely processed — homogenized, pasteurized and ultra-filtered. This is not raw milk!

Raw milk is an excellent example of a raw food which has the highest quality of complete protein. And we're not going to eat raw chicken, raw turkey, raw beef, or even raw eggs, (although raw eggs do make a delicious milk shake!). We also know that raw oysters are not going to be part of our daily diet, and wild oysters are becoming harder to come by. Milk has been a basic and very important dietary staple for thousands of years, and humans have thrived on it.

PASTEURIZATION

In the 1800s, humans caught typhoid and tuberculosis from tainted milk. Dairies in the 1800s were extremely unsanitary and so were the dairy workers. Tuberculosis and typhoid at the time were very common and easily spread. The solution invented to prevent these types of pandemics was to boil the milk. The problem with that? It tastes like boiled milk (let us assure you this is not a pleasant taste). As a result, a smart aleck by the name of Pasteur found that if you heated milk to just below the boiling temperature, you could kill 99.999 percent of the bacteria in the milk, and it didn't taste boiled. This process was aptly named Pasteurization.

Today the modern dairy industry is extremely sanitary and everything is sterilized with chlorine after each use. Nevertheless, the pasteurization process is used in almost all milk manufacturing.

The Pasteurization and Homogenization Pandemic

After commercialized farming became popular and it became common for cows to be fed primarily grains and even brewer's mash in overcrowded feedlots, people began to get sick from the milk. Rather than go back to the more natural way of process-

ing milk organically, which would cost too much, food manufacturers found that you could just pasteurize the milk and kill all the bad bacteria. Of course, it made it a very unhealthy milk, but at least it didn't make people sick from live disease-producing organisms. One of the major flaws of the pasteurization process is that pasteurization

The History of Milk

Approximately 10,000 years ago, milk cows were not fed cow feed, they got all of their food by grazing. Grains at that time were harvested by hand and were much too valuable to be fed to livestock.

As industry progressed, things like steam, diesel fuel, tractors, artificial fertilizers and modern farming equipment were invented. Suddenly, harvesting grains by modern farming methods became much easier and cheaper. This meant products like corn and grain were cheaper and more convenient than re-seeding fields that the livestock grazed on season after season. This meant that cows began to be herded to feedlots and fed corn and grains instead of being "free range." The grains fed were mostly corn-based and, corn having a higher protein content than grass and hay, meant larger cows who produced more milk (which also meant more money). This encouraged farmers to feed their cows more corn to get the cows to produce as much as five gallons of milk per day. This is great news for the farmers, right? Not necessarily. Unfortunately, disease spreads very easily in cattle feedlots. Since the milk was unpasteurized and unhomogenized (which was fine before the farming industry began using diesel fuels and fertilizers) and 100 percent organic, the disease spread to the milk.

does not remove bad bacteria, it just kills it, meaning the body still digests all the allergen-producing bacterial cells.

Pasteurization, according to the high-temperature short-time (HTST) method, requires milk to be heated to 161 F for 20 seconds. A quick inspection, however, of supermarket shelves revealed that there was no raw milk for sale. Most of the milk containers even had the words "Ultra-pasteurized" on the containers. The "Ultra" in ultra-pasteurized means that the milk has been heated to 280 F for less than a second. This is well above the boiling point of water.

Enzymes are specialized proteins that assist in the process of breaking down and digesting foods into nutrients so that they can be utilized, absorbed or stored by the body. For instance, *lipase* helps digest lipids (fats). *Lactase* helps digest lactose sugar (milk sugar). If your body does not produce and have available specific enzymes, then you may not be able to utilize certain food sources, or absorb certain minerals, etc. *Phosphatase* enzyme in milk, which is necessary for the absorption of calcium, is inactivated by pasteurization. In fact, the test for effective pasteurization is called the "negative phosphatase test." Is it no wonder that Americans are suffering from osteoporosis at a rate higher than ever. It is now considered a U.S. health crisis.

There are claims that milk produces mucous when you drink it. The production of mucous is an allergic reaction designed to clear away allergens. Milk is no more mucous producing than any other allergy-producing material, such as nuts, honey, shellfish, pet dander or any other allergen. For those who are allergic to cow's milk — don't drink it. There are people who are allergic to cow's milk that are not allergic to other types of milk. We recommend goat milk as an alternative to cow's milk.

The pasteurization process also destroys vitamin C. In a study, samples of raw milk, certified milk, certified Guernsey milk and certified vitamin D milk were collected at different dairies throughout the city of Madison, Wisconsin. These milks, on average, are only slightly lower in quality and nutrition than fresh milk, indicating that commercial raw and certified milks, as delivered to the consumer, lose only a small amount of their antiscorbutic potency. (Antiscorbutic ability is the ability to prevent scurvy. Scurvy is caused by the lack of ascorbic acid [vitamin C]).

Likewise, samples of commercial pasteurized milks were collected and analyzed. On average, they contained only about one-half as much ascorbic acid as fresh raw milks and significantly less ascorbic acid than the commercial unpasteurized milks. The following quote says it all.

"It was found that commercial raw milks contained an antiscorbutic potency, which was only slightly less than fresh raw milks and that pasteurized milks, on the average, contained only one-half the latter potency. Mineral modification and homogenization apparently have a destructive effect on ascorbic acid (Woessner[60]).

If left to stand or rest, good quality whole milk will separate into a creamy layer and a milky layer. For some reason, this has become unacceptable in the United States and the milk is "homogenized" to prevent this from happening. To achieve homogenization, the milk is violently pumped at high pressure through jets to break up the fat globules so that they can no longer rise to the top and are dispersed through the milk.

The problem with this process is that the fat now comes into contact with the enzymes in the milk and quickly becomes rancid. To prevent the milk from spoiling quickly, the milk is pasteurized to destroy the enzymes! Yes. You read it right — to destroy the enzymes. Now you have milk with no separable cream in it. Also, the beneficial bacteria, which makes lactase to digest the lactose, has been killed, and the phosphatase enzyme that helps absorb the calcium has been destroyed.

Raw milk has lactobacilli bacteria in it, which makes lactase enzyme in your intestines. This digests the lactose (McAfee[61]). That is why lactose intolerant people can drink raw milk who otherwise would have problems with pasteurized milk.

A clinical nutritionist and naturopath doctor named Geloff found that with thousands of patients, 8 out of 10 people who have a problem with milk do not have a problem when the milk is raw. *Lactose intolerance is not an allergy by a deficiency of lactase enzyme.* The cow is smart, it put plenty of lactase in the milk to help you digest lactose. Don't blame the cow, blame the process. *Pasteurization strips the milk of its natural lactase and nutrients.*

When you drive up California Highway 99 from Bakersfield to Fresno, you encounter huge dairy feedlots filled with cows wallowing in the mud and eating grain from a trough. No wonder the cows have to be given antibiotics and the milk has to be semi-cooked! The Holstein cows are so covered with mud that they look like Jerseys. Big Jerseys. Five miles before you get to the feedlot, the smell is already permeating the air.

Cows can be pastured with careful rotation so that they do not destroy the pasture, and they can be fed alfalfa when there is no pasture. A diet rich in grass and alfalfa would ensure healthier cows that produce healthier

An Alternate View

At times you may encounter peripheral arguments, such as cow's milk was meant for calves and not for humans. We can rebut that statement by stating tuna was meant for dolphins and not humans, and that berries were meant for birds. Some hard-core animal rights activists would argue that humans are stealing the milk from the calves and slaughtering the calves for veal. We would ask those activists if they would rather we turn the pasture into a cornfield and destroy hundreds of little animals, rabbits, voles, mice, quails, sparrows, doves, nesting birds and plants that live in the pasture. The best pastures have some tree shade, beneficial for nesting songbirds.

milk and healthier meat. However, this would require more time and energy from the farmers and, as we all know, time is money.

ORGANIC MILK

Some processors make organic homogenized pasteurized milk. The upside to this kind of milk is that it doesn't contain pesticides and hormones, however, the downside is that all the enzymes and beneficial bacteria still have been destroyed. Enzymes are enormously important to our bodies' functionality. They trigger activity in our bodies' organs, like dissolving fat, breaking down food into nutrients to be absorbed by the organs, renewing aging cells and providing your mind and body with new energy.

The absolute best option, if you can find it, is organic raw milk. If you are unable to find organic raw milk at your local grocery or market, check on the Internet for a source near you. Try Nature's, Trader Joe's or other health food stores. Many times these Natural markets can provide contact information to help you locate a local source. Also try milks such as Guernesy certified milk or certified vitamin D milk.

We have covered a lot of information in this chapter and you may be wondering how to put this information into practical use to fit your everyday life. We have compiled some raw recipes for you in Chapter 10 that are easy, quick, filling and nutritious — and they taste good! We don't expect you to convert to an all raw diet (although we wouldn't discourage it). We *do* encourage you to incorporate some raw foods each and every day into your diet. Do it for your overall health; to fight cancer; lower your risk of heart disease, diabetes and obesity; increase your energy; keep your digestive tract functioning properly and with regularity; and to just feel better every day.

One of our favorite recipes is the Watercress Berry Salad. You can find the recipe in Chapter 10.

Why Nature Knows Better Than the Food Manufacturers

CHAPTER 5

In Chapter 4, Why Raw Is Better, we showed how Nature made a perfect food, milk, and then how food manufacturers ruined it. We took the example of milk and showed that it is the perfect food, but only in the condition when it first leaves the udder.

Before pasteurization and homogenization, milk had lactose in it for energy and nature made provisions for lactase enzymes to be produced to digest the lactose. Milk had calcium in it and nature provided it with phosphatase enzyme to help the body absorb the calcium. Milk had vitamin C in it to boost the immune system and stimulate the body to make collagen fiber which makes bones and ligaments flexible and strong and to keep our arteries strong. Milk had beneficial bacteria in it, which suppressed the growth of harmful bacteria. The milk's fat was in globules (cream), which protected them from the enzymes in the milk.

So what did the food processors do? In one fell swoop they smashed the fat globules to smithereens (called homogenization) and destroyed the enzymes, vitamin C and bacteria by a process called ultra-pasteurization. Then they turned it into a white plastic liquid that can last for months on the shelves, which means more "bang for the buck" to consumers who want a product for their hard-earned money that will last for a long time.

We reiterate that whole, natural, unprocessed foods should always have priority above processed food. Getting more bang for our buck comes at a price infinitely higher than a few spoiled cups of milk — the price of our health and the health of our children, grandchildren and other loved ones. Is that a price you are willing to pay? Going raw or beginning the transition of adding raw foods into your diet is most definitely the way to go. However, in today's society where manufactured foods are overwhelmingly dominant, we are going to find, sooner or later, a package of food in our hands with a label on it. As long as you know what that label means, you can understand and use the information to make smart, informed choices.

In the United States, most packaged foods are required by law to list the nutritional facts of the food in plain sight on the product's packaging. This label gives us so much information in such a small space that even those of us who know what we are looking for have a hard time (especially if we are trying to focus on the label in a busy, harshly lit supermarket with our kids talking to us while we read). If you haven't seen a nutrition label before, it looks like this:

Nutrition Facts

Serving Size 1 cup (228g)
Servings Per Container 2

Amount Per Serving

	% Daily Value*
Total Fat 12g	**18%**
Saturated Fat 3g	**15%**
Trans Fat 3g	
Cholesterol 30mg	**10%**
Sodium 470 mg	**20%**
Total Carbohydrate 31g	**10%**
Dietary Fiber 0g	**0%**
Sigars 5g	
Protein 5g	
Vitamin A	**4%**
Vitamin C	**2%**
Calcium	**20%**
Iron	**4%**

To make reading that very important label a little easier, we have summarized some of the sections of the label and broken down the information so that you can know what information the food industry is trying to give you.

The most important part of the food label is the serving size. If the serving size is small, then the amount of calories stated on the label will also appear to be small. If the serving size is large, then the amount of protein may appear to be generous. To get the total amount of calories in the package, you have to multiply the amount of calories by the total number of servings per container. For instance, if there are 150 calories per serving in your can of soup, and there are 2.5 servings in the can, you are looking at 2.5 times 150, which equals 375 calories.

This applies to all nutritional information amounts listed on the label. It is very important to take the serving size into account. It is so easy to give a label a cursory review and think "oh, this is great, only 150 calories and 4 grams of fat — this is healthy and quick!" That would be correct if there is only one serving in the container. But what if there are four servings? Four times 150 is 600 calories and 16 grams of fat. This might not fit into your diet plan quite so easily, especially if you don't realize you will have eaten that many calories and planned your day around 150 calories and four grams of fat.

The daily calorie requirement for humans can vary from 1,500 to 3,000 calories per day, depending the size and the activity level of the person. If a person's daily calorie intake is exceeded, those excess calories will be turned into fat. If the daily calorie requirement is not met, your body will begin burning its existing fat supply, then turn to burning muscle for fuel. Because of this, it is extremely important to take in the proper amount of calories for either losing or maintaining weight.

FAT CALORIES

The nutrition label also indicates how many calories are contributed by fat (fat calories). This information is meant to give you, in our opinion, an unfounded cholesterol scare. To reduce aging caused by glycation from high blood glucose, it would be preferable to get your calories from fat, but not harmful trans fats. The fats you should consume, what you have probably heard referred to as "good fats" (like in avocados) should have the correct balance between omega-3 and omega-6 fatty acids. Unfortunately, this is NOT addressed by food labels. We will talk more about these "good fats" and "bad fats" a little later on.

DAILY VALUE PERCENTAGES (% DV)

The percent of daily value is an attempt to get you to control your fat, cholesterol and sodium intake. In this book we emphasize, instead, that you control your levels of important trace minerals, anti-oxidants, vitamins, enzymes, fiber and good fat intake with the correct omega-3 to omega-6 balance, as well as reducing daily carbohydrate intake (at least, to equal the daily calorie requirement). This, of course, includes the calories contributed by fat.

THE SALT STORY

There is much effort to demonize sodium (salt), but it must be pointed out that salt is an essential food for all animal life. Salt is essential for regulating the water and other fluids in our bodies. Salt is regulated by the kidneys, which determine how much sodium your body needs. Sodium can either be eliminated or retained depending on your body's individual needs for the day. In addition to regulating fluids, sodium is also important for brain function. The chloride is critically needed to make stomach acid (called hydrochloric acid) that then digests protein.

Exact chemical calculation indicates that the stomach needs one-third pound of salt to convert to acid to be able to digest one pound of protein. However, the body is able to recycle the sodium and chloride used up in the digestion process. So we don't quite need that exact amount to successfully digest the protein, especially since a lot of the proteins we consume have their own salt content.

You can ingest excessive amounts of sodium, however. Avoid this by eating plenty of fruits and vegetables, as they contain much more potassium than sodium.

LABEL CLAIMS: WHAT THEY REALLY MEAN

Food manufacturers promote their foods by making statements and claims on their labels. Here are some common claims along with our analysis of those claims. Some are catch-claims and phrases used to trick us into thinking we're eating healthy foods. Names and descriptions of some commonly found ingredients in our foods are also explained.

CLAIM: Natural, All Natural, 100-percent Natural

ANALYSIS: The term "All Natural," as opposed to "Organic," is not regulated in any way. While the United States Department of Agriculture (USDA) does have voluntary guidelines, such as: A natural product contains no "artificial" ingredient or added color and is only minimally processed. The label must also state what it means by natural, such as no artificial color or ingredients, minimally processed, etc. It remains that anybody can use a natural claim for any kind of food.

CLAIM: Contains Anti-oxidants.
ANALYSIS: The USDA allows manufacturers to claim anti-oxidant benefits if the serving contains at least 20 percent of the required daily value (RDV) of vitamin C, vitamin A and vitamin E, but if the claim is "good source of anti-oxidant beta-carotene," then at least 10 percent beta carotene must be present per serving and other forms of vitamin A make up the balance.

An anti-oxidant claim must also include the names of the nutrients that are the anti-oxidants. For example: "High in anti-oxidant vitamins C and E." However, it is possible for the label to include an asterisk or another type of symbol to indicate all the included anti-oxidants throughout the label. There are many other powerful anti-oxidants in foods, such as lycophene (contained in tomatoes and watermelons) and just because no anti-oxidant claim can be made for these, it does not mean there are no anti-oxidants present.

CLAIM: Cage Free, Free Range.
ANALYSIS: This claim is meaningless. The U.S. Department of Agriculture's definition of these terms in its entirety: "Producers must demonstrate to the Agency that the poultry has been allowed access to the outside." In other words, there has to be a door, and it has to be open at least part of the time. The size of the "outside" is not defined in any way, so technically, the chicken or turkey could have a one square-foot "yard" and it could be considered "Free Range, Cage Free."

CLAIM: Certified.
ANALYSIS: The term "certified" implies that the USDAs Food Safety and Inspection Service and the Agriculture Marketing Service have officially evaluated a meat product for class, grade or other quality characteristics (e.g., "Certified Angus Beef"). When used under other circumstances, the term must be closely associated with the name of the organization responsible for the "certification" process, (e.g., "XYZ Company's Certified Beef"). This means an inspector has found:
No.1: Yes, this sure looks like beef, carcass is too big to be a rabbit.
No. 2: Yes, it seems to have come from Angus cattle.
No. 3: The company has records.
No. 4: Yes, there are even some scared Angus cows outside.

CLAIM: Free (does not contain a specific item, e.g.: fat free, cholesterol free, sugar free).
ANALYSIS: FREE has hard and fast definitions set forth by the FDA.
Calorie free: Less than 5 calories per serving.
Cholesterol free: Less than 2 milligrams cholesterol and 2 grams or less saturated fat per serving.
Fat free: Less than 0.5 grams of fat per serving.
Sodium/salt free: Less than 5 milligrams per serving.
Sugar free: Less than 0.5 grams of sugars per serving.

CLAIM: High In (item of choosing).
ANALYSIS: Each serving must have at least 20 percent of the declared nutrient. For example, "High in fiber" means 2.5 to 4.9 grams

of fiber per serving and low in fat.

CLAIM: No Hormones, Hormone-free.
ANALYSIS: Pigs and chickens are not allowed to be given hormones, so this statement would be redundant. In the case of beef, the grower must merely be able to show documentation that no hormones were used in the raising of the animals. The meat actually isn't tested for hormones.

CLAIM: No Antibiotics.
ANALYSIS: This claim can be used for meat or poultry and the grower just has to provide documentation that no antibiotics have been given to the animals (via food, injection, or any other method).

CLAIM: Organic.
ANALYSIS: This is a legally defined and regulated term. The Organic Foods Production Act in the Federal code reads:
"Organic food is produced by farmers who emphasize the use of renewable resources and the conservation of soil and water to enhance environmental quality for future generations. Organic meat, poultry, eggs, and dairy products come from animals that are given no antibiotics or growth hormones. Organic food is produced without using most conventional pesticides; fertilizers made with synthetic ingredients or sewage sludge; bioengineering; or ionizing radiation. Before a product can be labeled 'organic,' a government-approved certifier inspects the farm where the food is grown to make sure the farmer is following all the rules necessary to meet USDA organic standards. Companies that handle or process organic food before it gets to your local supermarket or restaurant must be certified, too."

The code also has the entry: "Organic agriculture practices cannot ensure that products are completely free of residues; however, methods are used to minimize pollution from air, soil and water." This means that the farmer has some wiggle room if he has an insect infestation.

CLAIM: Kosher (and Halal).
ANALYSIS: Basically, the Kosher or Halal label means the food has been certified by a rabbi as conforming to Kosher, and Halal by a cleric conforming to Islamic laws. The kosher laws are very extensive and Wikipedia Encyclopedia gives a good account. In summary, though, you may only eat meat from animals that have cloven hooves and chew the cud, which means hare, hyrax, camel and pig are excluded. Halal is very similar to Kosher, except that Halal does not allow alcohol and other intoxicants, not even in skin cleansers.

Digestibility studies from a purely scientific point of view find that pork is more digestible than chicken (98 percent versus 95 percent) so the Kosher laws do not closely follow modern nutritional principles. Lobsters and oysters are super foods nutritionally, but are not allowed, especially oysters that are raw. Slaughter must include the removal of all the blood, as blood and fat are not allowed to be consumed.

CLAIM: Whole Wheat.
ANALYSIS: The term "Whole Wheat is allowed to be used on products that contain some whole wheat, but may also contain white flour, sugars, and other 'empty' ingredients. To ensure that refined flours are not present in the product, the label should state '100 percent whole wheat.' "

CLAIM: Hydrogenated Oils.

ANALYSIS: Hydrogenated oils are commonly found in mayonnaise, potato chips, cookies, crackers and most processed foods. We love all of those things, but they contain hydrogenated oils and trans fats. Hydrogenation

---

The Mayo Clinic, *http://www.mayoclinic.com*, defines fibromyalgia as a chronic condition characterized by widespread pain in your muscles, ligaments and tendons, as well as fatigue and multiple tender points (places on your body where slight pressure causes pain). Fibromyalgia occurs in about 2 percent of the population in the United States. Women are much more likely to develop the disorder than are men, and the risk of fibromyalgia increases with age. Fibromyalgia symptoms often begin after a physical or emotional trauma, but in many cases there appears to be no triggering event.

---

of oils turns unsaturated fats into saturated fats, so all omega fatty acids are destroyed. In addition, partial hydrogenation can convert its fatty acids into trans-fatty acids, which cannot be utilized by the body.

CLAIM: Refined Sugar.

ANALYSIS: Refined sugar is probably the biggest cause of disease in today's society. Refined sugar actually is a chemical called sucrose, which is a combination of glucose and fructose. Glucose causes glycation and fructose is an even more potent glycation agent. Glucose depresses the immune system by as much as 50 percent, which drastically reduces the body's resistance to infections and toxins. Although the sweetener Aspartame contains amino acids, phenylalanine and aspartic acid, which are naturally occurring, some people claim severe side effects from using it, including symptoms similar to celiac sprue (gluten allergy) and fibromyalgia.

Now that you are familiar with the food label and some of the most commonly used ingredients in processed foods, we encourage you to spend some time in your kitchen inventorying the foods you have and their nutritional values. If you have foods that are unhealthy or contain little or no nutritional value, donate them! If you leave them lurking in your cabinets, it becomes much easier to grab and eat, especially at the end of a long, stressful day. The best solution? Clear them out of your cupboard and out of your life. The best gift you can give yourself is good health and you are worth the time it takes to make these positive changes in your life. Trust us, if we can do it, you will have no problem.

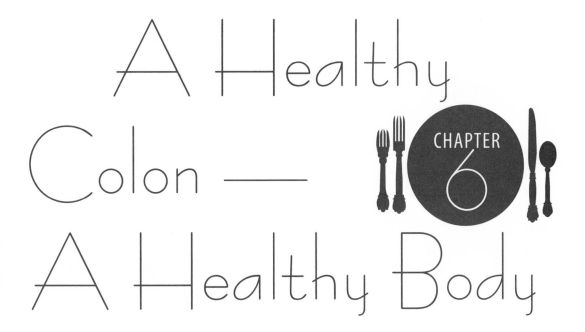

A Healthy Colon — A Healthy Body

CHAPTER 6

For some reason, the topics of digestive function, the colon, and bowl health have become an embarrassing topic, one that is only discussed under our breath and behind closed doors — if at all. Don't be embarrassed. Everybody talks about these issues. The stigma attached to discussing colon functions actually is pretty scary. It is scary because, if we are too nervous or embarrassed to talk about colon health, colon cancer, bowel function, and other digestive issues, then we might be too embarrassed to speak up when something feels wrong. Did you know that colorectal cancer, otherwise known as colon cancer, is the third most common cancer diagnosed in both men and women in the United States?

The American Cancer Society Web site states: "Colorectal cancer is the third leading cause of cancer-related deaths in the United States when men and women are considered separately, and the second leading cause when both sexes are combined. It was expected to cause about 49,920 deaths (25,240 in men and 24,680 in women) during 2009."

The numbers above show that we as a society have to stop being shy and start talking about our digestive health. Not only that, we must be proactive and take steps to make sure that our colon and bowels are clean, healthy, and working properly so that we can avoid becoming part of the statistic above.

The most critical component of our health and wellness is our digestive system, as we are entirely dependent on it to supply all of the water and food to our body (in the same way that we depend on our lungs to provide oxygen to our body). It is impossible to be healthy and free of disease if your digestive system is not functioning properly.

Bowel cleaning can be effective for helping relieve you from many ailments. Did you know that even back pain and headaches can be caused by a blocked, enlarged bowel? This is because the swollen bowel puts pressure on the spine, which causes tension and aches from the unexpected pressure. Every square inch of your abdomen is packed with something and there is just no room for anything else. If one organ swells, there is less room for the other organs. If the other organs become "squashed," they will send warning signals to your brain, which converts those signals into symptoms to draw your attention to the problem.

The digestive system of men and women in the United States has reached an all-time low in terms of health. Our digestive systems were designed to process natural, fiber-rich foods rich in protein, minerals and oils. The introduction of refined and processed foods with low fiber and high sugar content has wreaked havoc on our digestive systems. Disease such as colon cancer, diverticulitis, irritable bowel syndrome, polyps, constipation and sluggish bowel all have become rampant.

Diverticulitis

Diverticulitis, once almost unheard of, is now an amazingly common condition. Diverticulitis occurs when weak spots in the intestine bulge and trap food in pockets created by the bulge. The food trapped in those bulges becomes rotten because they are not broken down and expelled as your body intended. Many people have slight diverticulitis and never experience any symptoms, however, a great deal of people experience symptoms such as a tender lower abdomen (specifically on the left side), sudden and intense abdominal pain, cramping, nausea, and sudden constipation and/or diarrhea. These symptoms can vary from mild to intense and could be short-lived or increase slowly over a few days.

It is estimated that about 1 in 10 Americans over the age of 40, and over half of Americans over the age of 60, have diverticulitis. However, the percentage of people with diverticulitis under the age of 40 is rapidly increasing due to daily diets lacking in essential nutrients.

Bowel Movements

Because this topic is not one regularly discussed, most people have questions about what having "regular bowel movements" or "being regular" actually means. A normal, healthy bowel movement is a movement that is pain free and struggle free. The stool should be soft and easy to pass and should not be accompanied by cramping or bleeding. Medical doctors consider anything between one elimination per day to one elimination per week to be normal. However, Dr. Richard Schulze[62], who has helped thousands of people regain active healthy bowel action, disagrees. He studied people in nonindustrial countries that had a diet of unprocessed foods and found that they have two eliminations per day. They were quick, effortless and with soft light-colored, yet bulky, stools that were relatively odorless. Our goal should be to increase the fiber in our diet to achieve the same. Needless to say colon cancer was absent.

Luckily, a healthy bowel, colon and digestive tract can be achieved by simply eating right.

FOODS FOR BETTER BOWEL HEALTH

Below, we have listed some of the best foods and activities to help you become and stay regular and healthy.

Prunes

The bowel can be made to work more effectively with prunes, as they naturally help stimulate contractions of the intestines. Prunes can be eaten dried, blended (in a blender or juicer) with apple juice (make sure to soak them in water first to soften), or you can buy prune juice right off the shelves. If you choose to purchase prune juice, make sure that no sugar or corn syrup has been added.

Water

Water is critical to the proper function of the bowels and they cannot function effectively if you are dehydrated. Without enough water, waste cannot be effectively moved through the digestive track so it becomes hard and can even become lodged in the colon. This results in constipation and gas, both of which can be very painful. We recommend consuming at least two quarts of cold (or cool) unfluoridated water per day and more if you are very active.

Fiber

Fiber is the part of plant foods that absorbs water and pushes food through the intesti-

nal track, colon and bowels. Fiber also binds harmful acids in the small intestines, which makes them less likely to enter the blood stream. To get more fiber in our diet, we must eat more fruit, vegetables, grains, and sprouts. Vegetables in the cruciferous family are especially high in fiber and are most beneficial when eaten raw. In Chapter 10, we have included some delicious recipes rich in fiber that will help you get and stay regular.

Aloe Vera

Similar to prunes, aloe vera increases the strength and number of contractions of the intestines. It also loosens and discharges undigested food bacteria and parasites that stick to the colon.

The most reliable way to obtain an active form of aloe vera is to make it fresh from aloe leaves. To do this, you will need fresh aloe plants, which can be purchased from a nursery. With a sharp knife, carefully remove the skin from the inner gel. Eating the inner gel has an amazing cleaning effect on the gut. It is important to remove all of the skin, as it contains a bitter sticky yellow material that can be irritating to the intestinal linings. To cleanse the bowel, consume two 8 oz. glasses of aloe per day for five days.

If you don't have time to find aloe plants and skin them, aloe vera can be purchased from health food stores or markets and even at some farmers markets. When purchasing aloe vera, bear in mind that it can easily be inactivated by improper processing. Purchase aloe products that have the IASC seal on it, which is a green aloe plant on a white background with the word "certified" underneath. This certification means it has been tested and found to comply with the International Aloe Science Council, Inc. standards. A list of certified aloe products can be found on the IASC Web site: *www. IASC.org.*

Tips for Adding Fiber-Rich Foods Into Your Diet

Including fiber in your diet, staying hydrated, exercising, and performing occasional bowel cleanses are all important pieces in achieving a healthy, clean body. If, after following the directions in this chapter, you are still having digestive problems, please talk to your doctor. Don't let a few moments of talking about a subject that may be a little uncomfortable come between you and your health. Here's a few suggestions to get started:

Add fresh fruit to your breakfast cereal or whip them into pancake batter.

Snack on fresh, chopped raw vegetables like broccoli, cauliflower, carrots, and bell peppers. For an added treat, dip your fresh veggies in hummus.

Substitute black beans or pinto beans for refried beans at restaurants.

Use whole-grain pastas and breads instead of white.

Add sprouts to your salads and sandwiches.

Make kabobs with lean meat, bell peppers, onions, garlic, and pineapple. By baking the kabobs instead of grilling, you will keep the anti-cancer and anti-heart disease compounds in the vegetables alive.

Use whole-wheat English muffin halves to make mini-pizzas. Top with tomato sauce, fresh mozzarella cheese and your choice of vegetables (we prefer green bell peppers and onions).

Try something new! Cactus is a great source of fiber and it tastes great. You can find cooking directions and many recipes online.

Plantago Psyllium (Plantain)

Plantain seed husks expand and become mucilaginous when wet, especially those of Plantago psyllium, which is used in common over-the-counter bulk laxative and fiber supplement products such as Metamucil®. Plantago psyllium seed is used to relieve symptoms of conditions such as constipation, irritable bowel syndrome and diverticulitis. Plantain has been consumed as human food since prehistory. Psyllium supplements are typically used in powder form along with adequate amounts of fluids. There are a number of psyllium products used for constipation. The usual dose is about 3.5 grams twice a day. Psyllium is also a component of several ready-to-eat cereals.

Oregon Grape Root

Initially disagreeable to those not familiar with bitter herbs, Oregon grape root has a beneficial effect on the digestive tract. It stimulates the flow of bile, which loosens the stools and helps prevent and sometimes relieve constipation, diverticulitis, gallbladder disease and hemorrhoids. It may also help people with constipation-predominant irritable bowel syndrome (IBS).

Oregon grape root also has antibiotic and anti-cancer properties that are receiving more and more attention by researchers and clinicians. Berberine and other alkaloids have been shown to kill a wide range of microbes and have been effective in human studies for speeding recovery from giardia, candida, viral diarrhea, and cholera.

Studies in China show that it contains

an alkaloid named berbamine, which helps protect bone marrow and promotes its recovery from chemotherapy and radiation therapy for cancer. Combined with its bitter digestive-strengthening properties, Oregon grape root has an interesting and distinctive combination of properties.

Oregon grape root is taken either as a tea or tincture. To make tea, simmer one to two teaspoons of dried, coarsely chopped root in one cup of water for 10 to 15 minutes. Strain out the leftover root (or eat it, if you prefer), and sip the remaining liquid just before eating each substantial meal.

A tincture is an alcohol extract of the root. To make, mix one-half to one teaspoon of the purchased tincture in two to four ounces of water and sip before each meal. The amount of alcohol in tinctures at this dose is very low and presents no significant problem.

Senna

Senna is a plant that has leaves and pods containing compounds called anthraquinones. Anthraquinones are very powerful laxatives and should never be used by children or pregnant or nursing women. Senna should also never be used for more than seven consecutive days.

While we do not recommend using senna (aloe vera is milder and very effective), you can find it in capsule, tablet, or liquid forms. If you decide to try senna, please do so carefully and talk with your doctor before taking it.

Cascara Sagrada

Cascara sagrada is the dried bark of the cascara buckthorn, a small deciduous tree. The dried bark contains emodin, a substance that, when it comes into contact with the bowel, causes the bowel to contract. Medical students have found that it will even cause the bowel of dead people to contract. The act of causing the muscle to move also strengthens the muscle, just like in the gym where using your muscles strengthens them.

Exercise

All exercise increases peristaltic muscle waves, that's the muscular contraction of the bowel. Just like any other muscle, a lack of daily exercise results in weakness. If your intestinal muscles are weak, they are not able to contract strongly enough to push waste through them, especially not if you are dehydrated and the waste has become too large or too hard. To keep your digestive system muscles toned and working properly, we recommend, at minimum, at least 30 minutes of exercise five days per week.

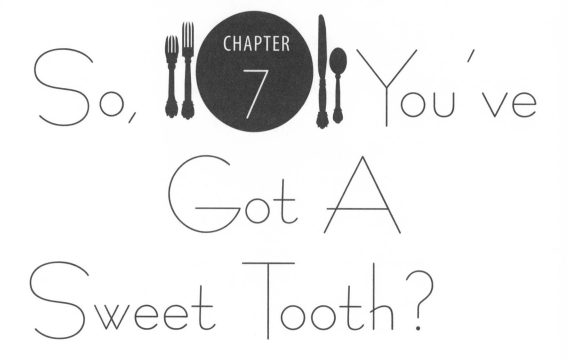

So, You've Got A Sweet Tooth?

CHAPTER 7

Our white blood cells are responsible for fighting infection in our body and antibiotics are not what the body normally uses to fight disease. No disease-producing organism can resist destruction by properly functioning white blood cells, but these organisms can easily build up a resistance to antibiotics and vaccines. The white blood cells in our bodies fail to destroy disease-producing organisms because the white blood cells do not have sufficient access to vitamin C. Vitamin C is the fuel that white blood cells use to destroy organisms and diseased cells. The more severe the infection, the larger amount of vitamin C needed, as much as 10,000 milligrams of vitamin C is required for life-threatening infections. Our bodies cannot make vitamin C, so we must get it from our diet or by supplementation.

Glucose also destroys the white blood cell's ability to fight disease, which is why people who consume a lot of carbohydrates and sugar have weak immune systems. As humans, one of the greatest hindrances to our immune systems is our excess sugar intake. White sugar looks innocent and tastes great, and can really satisfy our sweet tooth, but the price is much too high. White sugar can cause diabetes, depress the immune system, even make you look older (anything but that!).

In this chapter, we will teach you how to become immune from infectious disease by the use of a simple nutrient. This nutrient occurs in fruit, berries and vegetables. It is all-natural, fights infection, and removes foreign substances from the body. Curious? Keep reading!

INFECTIOUS DISEASES

In previous chapters, we taught you the natural way to overcome the biggest diseases of civilization, namely: heart disease, cancer and arthritis. By merely reverting our diet back to the way Nature intended, we can become healthier. However, we have yet to talk about one serious health factor — infectious disease.

Infectious diseases are pneumonia, flu (regular and pandemic), tuberculosis, colds, tooth abscesses, bleeding gums, boils, blood poisoning, hepatitis, meningitis, polio and any viral or bacterial disease. Even though each of these diseases are very different from each other, we group them together as they all are infectious. We do this simply because the body uses the same procedure to rid itself from all of these infections.

Medical science is limited to the use of antibiotics and vaccines that can be ineffective and do very little, if anything, to help the natural infection-fighting process in the body. Because of the constant mutation of infections, new antibiotics and vaccines have to be continually developed to deal with pathogens that have become resistant to the antibiotics already in use. In addition, antibiotics are not effective for curing viruses, although some doctors still prescribe them even though they will not cure or stop the virus.

Why would a doctor prescribe a medication that will not cure what ails you? Because taking antibiotics will not hurt you and antibiotics are a big source of revenue. Pharmaceutical companies love antibiotics and vaccines because manufacturing them is very cheap and they are sold in mass quantities — big profit earners for drug companies.

Time for the good news! No antibiotic or vaccine can compete with the most powerful infection fighter that exists — your body.

In each of our bodies we have things called "phagocytes." You probably are more familiar with their common name, white blood cells. As opposed to antibiotics, which are only good for fighting one particular pathogen, white blood cells don't discriminate. Whatever pathogen they find (if it is foreign to the body), the white blood cells destroy. The cells do this by surrounding the germ like an envelope and digesting it, thereby eradicating it. White blood cells are so strong they can even seek out and destroy tumor cells and debris inhaled into your lungs.

INFECTION-FIGHTING WHITE BLOOD CELLS

If white blood cells are so good at destroying infections, why do we still get them? The answers are very simple. Our white blood cells are starved of nutrition because of our unnatural diets. Because they are starving, they are not able to work at optimum capacity. Just like we are not going to function at full capacity if we have a sleepless night and then don't eat breakfast in the morning. Also a detriment is excessive sugar and carbohydrate intake, which poison and paralyze the white blood cells.

The most critical nutrient the white bloods cell needs in order to function properly is vitamin C, and the more work the white blood cells need to do, the more vitamin C they need. Think of vitamin C as the gasoline that fuels the white blood cells. If we have only a few bacteria in our body to destroy, the white blood cells are quite happy to use a small amount of vitamin C.

However, if we have a massive and/or life-threatening infection, the white blood cells need massive amounts of vitamin C. If we have insufficient vitamin C in our bodies, the white blood cells are overcome and too weak to deal with the threat. With an unlimited supply of vitamin C, the white blood cells become like an army of super heroes, destroying all the germs and, in effect, saving our lives. This is a pretty miraculous process and it happens every single day of our lives.

THE LACK AND BENEFITS OF VITAMIN C

All animals can make vitamin C from the sugar contained in their livers. The more vitamin C the body needs, the more the animal can make. However, we humans have a genetic defect that prevents us from making our own vitamin C. The mechanism is there, it just doesn't work like it does in animals. The liver cannot make the enzyme *L-gulonolactone oxidase* that is responsible for making vitamin C. This means we are responsible for getting enough vitamin C to support our bodies exclusively from food or supplements.

Unfortunately, vitamin C is very unstable and is easily lost from our foods. The simple act of cooking destroys most of the vitamin C contained in our foods and, if our diet is lacking in raw fruit and vegetables, we hardly get any vitamin C. Sadly, it is pretty safe to say that all of us are vitamin C deficient.

The insulin in our bodies causes vitamin C to move into our cells, including white blood cells. As much as 80 times more vitamin C has been found in white blood cells than in blood plasma. Once the vitamin C enters the white blood cells, it stimulates the production of something called

*nicotinamide adenine dinucleotide phosphate-oxidase (*NADPH). NADPH is made from niacin (vitamin B3). The NADPH then has the ability to make hydrogen peroxide, the same material that is sold over the counter as a germ killer or to bleach your hair. The hydrogen peroxide kills, digests and destroys all bacteria, even tumor cells, that are engulfed by the white blood cells.

How Much is Enough?

Each and every person has a different level of need for vitamin C, so it virtually is impossible to tell how much vitamin C per day is needed on a person by person basis. One person may need only 100 milligrams per day whereas another person with a serious health challenge may need 15 grams. The person who needs only a dose of 100 milligrams per day on a regular basis, may need a dose of 4 grams if they start coming down with the flu. The body also may accept a lot of vitamin C if the bones and ligaments have been weakened by a history of vitamin C deficiency. This is because vitamin C is also needed to make collagen, which strengthens the bones (and fights wrinkles). Dr. Schep took two grams a day for two years at the age of 56 to get his bones strong in preparation for playing rugby. Only after two years did he begin to get overdose symptoms (diarrhea).

Generally speaking, most young, healthy people should be okay with a daily vitamin C intake of anywhere from 60 to 100 milligrams a day. In the following circumstances, a person would need the noted vitamin C amounts. Using these guidelines, most minor to moderate infections will disappear within 24 to 48 hours.

Common cold: 2 to 4 grams every four

hours until cold lessens.

Flu : 4 grams every four hours until fever disappears.

Tooth abscess: 4 grams every four hours until pain and swelling are gone.

Hepatitis: 4 grams every four hours until cured (usually within one to two days).

Cancer: 10 to 15 grams per day or as much as the body will tolerate.

To determine your daily vitamin C requirement, keep increasing your vitamin C intake. When your body has enough vitamin C it will reject the excess by causing diarrhea. At that point you can cut back, confident that you are healthy and have sufficient C (and a clean colon!).

Foods Rich In Vitamin C

Although we can boost our immune system tremendously with supplements such as vitamin C powders, tablets and pills, thereby enhancing a natural process, the most natural form of vitamin C is that which we can get from our food. The foods that we consume (or should be consuming) have vitamin C occurring simultaneously with other anti-oxidants like polyphenols and bioflavonoids. Together with vitamin C, these anti-oxidants fight disease, give you energy and keep you strong and healthy.

The richest vitamin C food is Rose hips. Rose hips can be eaten raw or you can purchase dried hips from a health store and use them to make tea. Rose hips contain anywhere from 1,000 to 2,500 milligrams of vitamin C per 100 grams, depending on variety.

Barbados cherries, also known as acerola, contains approximately 1,700 milligrams of vitamin C per 100 grams. You can purchase acerola powder from a health food store or you can grow your own if you live in a climate similar to that of Florida or Hawaii (or if you have a large hot house).

The table below lists other foods that are rich in vitamin C.

SUGAR — THE SAD TRUTH ABOUT THE SWEET TREAT

Insulin causes cells not only to absorb ascorbic acid, but also glucose. Unfortunately, when glucose enters the white blood cells, it lessens the ability of the white blood cells to make NADPH. That means less hydrogen peroxide is produced, which makes the body's immune system performance tank. It's estimated that the average person's immune system is reduced to half of its effectiveness due to daily sugar intake. Half! No wonder the average person's immunity to diseases is

FOOD NAME	SERVING SIZE	VITAMIN C CONTENT
Blackcurrant	100 grams	155 milligrams
Kiwi fruit	100 grams	100 milligrams
Redcurrant	100 grams	58 to 80 milligrams
Papaya	100 grams	62 milligrams
Strawberry	100 grams	57 milligrams
Orange	100 grams	53 milligrams

114

so poor. Our high sugar intake and low vitamin C intake are allowing rampant cancer and infectious diseases, as the white blood cells are unable to destroy cancer cells or bacteria if they're overloaded with glucose. And it's not just sugar; carbohydrates produce blood glucose too (A. Sanchez[63]).

It is almost impossible to purchase any kind of processed food without sugar or high-fructose corn syrup. Due to our unhealthy diets and the addition of high-fructose corn syrup (which is 50 percent glucose!), it is estimated that sugar consumption per citizen in the United States has gone up from a few pounds a year to 155 pounds per person — per year. Next time you are at the grocery store, swing by the baking aisle and take a look at the shelf of one-pound sugar cartons or bags. Envision how eating 155 of those cartons per year would make you feel. Awful, right? But this is exactly what we are doing each and every year and, by doing so, we are slowly killing ourselves.

Dr. Nancy Appleton has done much research on the effects of sugar in the body. In her research, she has found information from hundreds of scientific papers[64] supporting the following facts about sugar:

Suppresses the immune system.

Upsets mineral deficiencies.

Interferes with absorption of calcium.

Causes anxiety.

Causes hyperactivity.

Causes difficulty concentrating and moodiness in children (causes a rapid rise in adrenaline).

Promotes the loss of tissue elasticity and function.

Feeds cancer cells.

Increases fasting levels of glucose.

Weakens eyesight.

Speeds up premature aging.

Interferes with protein digestion.

Enlarges the liver.

Enlarges kidneys.

Increases fluid retention.

Makes tendons brittle.

Reduces learning capacity.

Lessens circulation.

Slows down adrenals.

Increases polio risk.

In addition, hundreds of papers showed moderate to high sugar consumption promotes the following diseases:

Bowel disease
Alcoholism
Periodontal disease
Cavities
Obesity
Arthritis
Asthma
Multiple sclerosis
Yeast infections
Gallstones
Appendicitis
Hemorrhoids
Varicose veins
Osteoporosis
Diabetes
Blood pressure
Food allergies
Toxemia during pregnancy
Eczema
Emphysema
Cataracts and nearsightedness
Migraines
Depression
Gout
Dizziness
Epileptic seizures
Gum disease

SUGAR ALTERNATIVES

The best alternative to sugar is no sugar at all. Easier said than done, right? If you just have to have real sugar, it must only be a very small amount — less than two teaspoons per day.

The good news is you don't have to give up sweets! Mother Nature has provided us some delicious, healthy alternatives to highly refined white sugar and high-fructose corn syrup. The absolute best alternative is *blackstrap molasses*. Blackstrap molasses actually is a super food, as it contains all the minerals (copper, iron, manganese and selenium) that fight serious diseases such cancer, arthritis, obesity and heart disease. These minerals are highly concentrated due to the process that is used to remove them from the sugar cane juice. Our second preference is dark maple syrup, which can easily be found in the health food section of your supermarket or in your local natural foods store. We recommend using dark maple syrup to sweeten your coffee or tea and using blackstrap molasses to sweeten your cereal or oatmeal.

Another delicious and natural way to sweeten teas, water (flat and sparkling), baked goods, syrups and more is to use fresh fruit juice (unpasteurized wherever possible). Not only do the juices taste good and add new dimensions, they also contain antioxidants such as carotene and vitamin C.

For baking, we recommend using *stevia* in the place of sugar as it is a completely natural plant material. The stevia plant actually has a history of use as a medicinal plant amongst tribal people. For centuries, South American tribes used it as sweetener in yerba mate (a popular stimulant drink that is similar to tea) and it is used in me-

dicinal teas for treating heartburn and other ailments. More recent medical research has even shown promise in treating obesity and hypertension with stevia. In addition, stevia has a negligible effect on blood glucose, even enhancing glucose tolerance. It's an attractive natural sweetener for diabetics and others on carbohydrate-controlled diets.

The following are sweeteners to replace unhealthy white sugar.

Maple Syrup (Not to be Confused With Pancake Syrup)

Use the darkest syrup you can find; it is more concentrated and has more minerals. Use three-fourths cup of maple syrup for one cup sugar and decrease the total amount of liquid in the recipe by three tablespoons for each cup of syrup that you use.

Stevia

Stevia goes a long way, so use moderately. One-half teaspoon stevia extract is the same sweetness as one cup of sugar. It does not work with yeast-risen breads, so use with quick-rising recipes. Stevia powder also works well with citrus flavors so it's good in lemonade, etc.

Date Sugar

Date sugar simply is finely ground dates so it does not have the melting quality of sugar. It goes through minimal processing which makes it more healthy. Baking with it will cause the color of your baked goods to become darker. It is suggested that you use two-thirds cup date sugar to substitute one cup of sugar. We suggest you use date sugar to sprinkle on yogurt or on cinnamon toast.

Grape Molasses

An exceptionally delicious molasses, it is a good source of calcium, iron, potassium and magnesium with lots of other minerals. Try tahini and grape molasses; one-half the amount of molasses to tahini and mix until well blended. Spread on bread instead of using peanut butter and jelly. Use grape molasses to sweeten a vinaigrette pour over raw spinach and pine nuts. Grape molasses can be found in Greek or Mediterranean stores or possibly your local health food store.

Unsulfered Blackstrap Molasses (Known as Treacle in Europe)

This molasses has a very strong flavor. We suggest you use it as recommended in a recipe calling for blackstrap molasses. To substitute for one cup of sugar, try using one-half cup blackstrap molasses and one-half cup maple syrup. Reduce the liquid content by three tablespoons (some say five tablespoons). You'll have to experiment since there are not many recipes available without white flour when it comes to baking and using alternative sweeteners. Try two tablespoons blackstrap molasses in your coffee. It is a powerful source of the critical minerals, copper and manganese, missing in our diets.

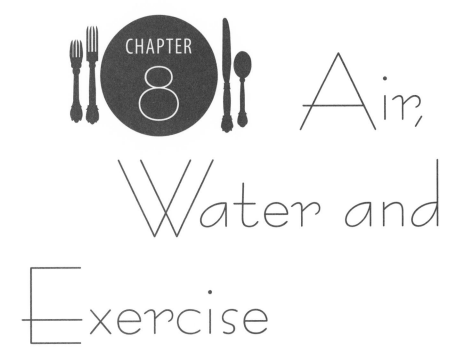

Air, Water and Exercise

Fresh air, water and exercise are basic rights for everyone. Are you taking full advantage of these rights? By just increasing your daily intake of water you will improve your skins elasticity, decrease or eliminate muscle cramps, and kick start your metabolism. By doing something as simple as breathing correctly, you will increase blood flow to your body and brain, reduce muscle tension, and increase mental clarity.

AIR

The most important substance needed for health and for life is air, as we cannot live without it for more than a few minutes. The air we breathe has the important function of supplying oxygen to our cells so that fuel can be burned to produce heat and energy. Air also has the function of carrying the carbon dioxide and water out of our bodies that is produced by combustion.

Since we are so critically dependant on air, it is important to make sure we take the time to breathe properly. Without proper breathing, you tend to feel sluggish, forgetful and tense (sound familiar?). In fact, most people don't breathe properly.

Tune Up Your Lungs for the Indy 500 of Life

To fully benefit from proper breathing, our lungs must be fit and healthy and in top working condition. When the air enters our nose, it goes into the trachea and down to the bronchial tubes into the air sacs, which are called *alveoli*. All of these body parts must be elastic to expand and contract appropriately. The prime nutrient for elasticity is — wait for it — Copper! Copper is part of the *lysyl oxidase* enzyme, which makes elastin tissue.

The nose, not the mouth is designed for air intake. If the nose is blocked or stuffy due to colds, then the vitamin C intake must be dramatically increased to get rid of the cold causing the stuffiness so the body can resume its natural way of breathing.

When we inhale, dirt, dust and debris must be removed from the lungs. The mucous membranes contain *villi* which help move debris particles up and out of the lungs where they can either be swallowed or expelled (coughed up). Therefore coughing performs an extremely important function, namely that of cleaning out your lungs. Smaller particles of solids, including bacteria, are engulfed by white blood cells.

To ensure proper health of our respiratory system, we need the following:

Vitamin A: For mucous membrane health (carrots are an excellent source of vitamin A).

Iron: For red blood cell health (to optimize the transfer of oxygen to the red blood cells).

Omega-3 oil: Mediates excessive inflammation in the lungs, which can cause reduced air supply.

The use of artificial anti-inflammatories will not address the cause — lack of omega-3.

Poor Breathing Effects

Proper breathing is important to everyone, but those living in high-altitude locations need to be especially diligent in practicing proper breathing techniques. The higher you are in altitude, the less oxygen there is in the space surrounding you.

If you are breathing improperly, you are not getting a complete supply of oxygen. When our oxygen supply is incomplete, the body increases the supply of blood to your brain, as lack of oxygen can cause brain damage. Since the heart is pumping a larger supply of blood to the brain than normal, it then decreases the supply of blood to the rest of your body (poor circulation). If the brain still is not getting enough oxygen, mild to moderate impairment of brain function can occur. The impairment generally is mild but creates symptoms such as difficulty with complex learning tasks, loss of clarity and focus, reduced motivation and short-term memory loss.

In prolonged situations of poor oxygen supply to the brain, more serious symptoms such as fainting can occur. Luckily, these symptoms are rare and, more often than not, curable by proper breathing.

Proper At-Rest Breathing Techniques

The lungs start just below the shoulders and continue right down to the diaphragm (which is just above the stomach). Nature intended for the entire lung to be used for breathing, but most people just suck air into the top half of their lungs by moving their chest. When we do that, the air in the bottom half of our lungs becomes stale and useless.

The proper way to breath is with your stomach. This sounds a little odd, but try this: Stand up or sit up straight and inhale deeply through your nose. You should feel the entire area between the chest and your lower abdomen expand. When you exhale, you should feel your stomach pulling back in as you empty the air from your lungs. This probably will feel a little strange at first and it definitely takes some concentration in the beginning. If you do this breathing exercise a few times each day and quicken the process each time you do it, it will fast become the normal, thoughtless way you breathe. Proper breathing when you are exercising becomes even more important so that your lungs and cardiovascular system can function at optimum capacity.

When you wake up in the morning, you are probably the most oxygen starved. You can flood your body with life-giving oxygen — no hyperbaric chamber needed — by taking about six very deep breaths outside (if possible). Inhale deeply, feeling your stomach and abdomen push outward. Hold the breath in as long as you comfortably can and then exhale completely, feeling your stomach and abdomen pull back in toward your spine. This invigorating routine floods the brain and body with oxygen, giving your body the fuel it needs to wake up and function well. This practice is common for people who practice sunrise yoga. In sunrise yoga, seven deep breaths is the norm.

WATER

Outside of the air we breathe, the second most critical life-giving substance we need is water. We can survive for weeks without food but only days without water. This is because our brains are 95 percent water, blood is 82 percent water and our lungs are 90 percent water.

A mere 2 percent drop in our body's water supply can trigger signs of dehydration such as fuzzy memory, trouble with math, and difficulty focusing on small print. It is generally recommended we get eight glasses of water a day (a glass equaling eight ounces). This is a total of 64 ounces or half

Hyperbaric Therapy (HBT)

Hyperbaric therapy is based on the principle that if you increase the pressure of air, then more oyxgen is taken up by the lungs. This is why you find it harder to breathe and exercise at very high altitudes. It involves the use of a chamber that can be sealed with you inside and the air pressure increased. This then increases the amount of oxygen in the blood, brain and spinal fluid, allowing the cells in your body greater access to oxygen, and thereby allow them to perform better, thereby resulting in improved health. The Yogis have known about this for thousands of years and are able to increase their blood oxygen supply by breathing exercises instead.

a gallon daily. However, your daily water requirement can vary considerably depending on your daily activity level, the climate you live in and other outside factors like performing hard work or exercise in high temperatures. Thirst is our best guide, if our thirst requires us to drink more, or less, than the recommended amount, this should be our guide. If you feel hungry more often than normal, you may be starting to get dehydrated. Drink a glass of water and wait 10 minutes or so. If you are still hungry, it really is hunger. If not, your body was just in need of hydration.

Water and Our Body

Sixty-four ounces of water seems like an awful lot of fluid, but our body really does need large quantities of water to operate at its maximum capacity and perform the following functions:

Causes of Dehydration

Not drinking enough water.
Excessive sweating due to heat and exercise.
Blood loss.
Vomiting.
Diarrhea.
Malnutrition.
Excessive alcohol intake (diuretic affect).
Excessive salt intake (the body must maintain the correct balance between salt and water).

Flush toxins out of the body through the kidneys.

Cool the body by means of sweating when it gets overheated (via exercise, sun exposure, fever, etc.).

Create saliva to aid digestion (especially if you eat dry or salty foods).

Alleviate constipation by moving food through the intestinal tract and eliminating waste.

Lubricate our joints.

Sufficient water can even dilute carcin-ogens by diluting them and flushing them out of our colon, bladder, kidneys and liver.

In a small way, water is even a source of trace elements for the body, such as sodium, chloride, calcium and magnesium.

Dehydration

Usually when we think of dehydration, we think of chapped lips, tiredness, dry skin or the lethargic feeling during a fever. We also tend to think of dehydration only when we are sick or when we have been exposed to severe temperatures for a few hours. The truth of the matter is, over 80 percent of humans are at least slightly dehydrated every single day.

Dehydration can occur when your body fluid levels are 2 percent less than what your body requires. The introduction of diet colas, energy drinks and salty, chemical-laden food has had a major impact on the amount of water we consume and retain. A 2 percent drop in water is a large enough drop to significantly lower the amount of blood your body has to circulate. A drop of 5 percent means you have much less blood circulating than your body requires as the blood becomes thicker and moves slower.

The following are dehydration symptoms to be mindful of. If you begin to experience any of the symptoms, start slowly hydrating immediately.

Increased thirst.

Appetite loss (due to less water in the stomach).

Dry skin.

Dark urine (this happens because your body has less water to flush toxins).

Dry mouth is a lack of saliva.

Fatigue and weakness (the less water, the less blood, which brings oxygen and glucose to your muscles.

Severe muscle cramps.

Chills and shivering (means insufficient blood to bring heat to the extremities of your body).

Light headed or dizzy upon standing (means not enough blood to your brain due to lack of water).

Mental fatigue, mental exhaustion and sleepiness (means less blood to bring oxygen and nutrients to your brain).

If you experience any of these symptoms, you know what to do — drink water! The best form of water is pure water, not sports or caffeinated beverages, as pure water is the best for cleansing the kidneys.

Types of Water: Good and Bad

Amazingly, nature supplies you with the right kind of water depending on your environment. If you live in the arid desert, the water naturally tends to be brackish. This means that the water naturally has a high salt content. This is due to the high evaporation rate of the water source (river, stream, other body of water). This water can also supply you with more electrolytes needed for high desert heat.

Freshly melted snow water in cold climates has little salt, which is just fine for the body when it is cold, but would not be the best type of water for someone enjoying a hot Arizona summer.

Distilled water and water that has been purified by reverse osmosis are the least beneficial to your body, even though they are the two most advertised and available types of water on the market. We say this because artificial distilled water does not occur in nature. The same applies for water purified by reverse osmosis, which is sold as "purified water." Think of our forefathers again, they drank water directly from unpolluted streams, lakes and rivers, getting minerals and nutrients necessary for proper body function.

Tap water is undesirable because it has been "enhanced" with fluoride. Fluoride is a harmful poison when ingested. Tap water also has gone through the chlorination process, which introduces chloroform and other halogenated substances into the water.

Water has organic substances in it, picked up from the mud, leaves and river banks as it flows. These organic substances are called humic acids. When the water is chlorinated, the chlorine reacts with these organic humic acids and bromide in the water to form chloroform and bromoform. These substances have been shown to generate free radicals in the liver. This increases the chance of cells turning cancerous, especially if we have low levels of superoxide dismutase (SOD) activity in our livers due to copper and manganese deficiency.

Mountain spring water is the best for you, as it comes into contact with rocks deep in the earth, extracting trace elements and minerals as it flows. Some mineral springs produce water so highly mineralized that it is bottled and sold as a health drink. France and Germany, in particular, sell the most brands of mineral water, but the USA also has a wide variety of available brands that are sold in grocery stores, upscale markets and drugstores.

When choosing a bottle of water, preferably a bottle of mountain spring water, choose a glass bottle if possible. Plastics can contaminate the water with the chemical that the plastic is made from, called the "monomer." Monomers can be toxic and should not be consumed. If a plastic bottle or container becomes warm, it slightly expands and monomer "leaks" or "fumes" into the contents of the bottle.

Sports Drinks

Sports drinks, although generally sold in plastic bottles, can be beneficial as they replace electrolytes in the body. The ideal "stats" for an eight-ounce sports drink: Sodium: 110 to 220 milligrams; carbohydrates: 14 to 20 grams per 8 ounces; mineral content: copper and iron.

Sports drinks ideally should contain copper, which supports the cardiovascular system and iron, which supplies more oxygen to the cells. The amount of copper and iron may be limited by the metallic taste it would give the drink, but even a small amount is greatly beneficial.

Higher amounts of carbohydrates are not recommended as something too sweet can cause thirst instead of quenching it. Unfortunately, we were not able to find any sports drinks on the market that contained copper and/or iron, but hopefully sports drink manufacturers eventually will include them in their formulas.

If at all possible, avoid sports drinks that have artificial coloring in them, as these are synthetic substances and not beneficial for the human body. Since the body doesn't need the synthetic substances it has to eliminate them. Doesn't sound too bad, but remember, you are drinking to hydrate, not to eliminate.

During athletic training, the exercise stimulates the formation of *human growth hormone* (HGH). Studies have found if you are dehydrated during training, this lessens the ability of the body to make HGH, although proper recovery is critical. This is great news for people suffering from joint pain who are paying through the roof for HGH injections. Sports drinks containing protein can be used for recovery after exertion and have been found to significantly lessen muscle soreness and cramping. On page 180 you will find a great recipe for an excellent, totally natural, raw, fresh protein drink recipe that helps increase human growth hormone (HGH) in the body.

Red Wine

A nice glass of wine paired with a lean healthy dinner can be the perfect way to wind down after a long day. What you might not know is that the red color in wine comes from *resveratrol*, which is a potent anti-aging compound that also prevents heart disease. Pinot Noir has almost twice the amount of resveratrol as most of the other reds.

Red wine is also rich in flavonoids, the same anti-oxidants that are found in fruits like oranges and apples. Wine also benefits from its glass bottling; you need not worry about monomer consumption.

As with any alcohol, drink responsibly and moderately, but enjoy the benefits of younger looking skin and a healthy heart while doing so!

EXERCISE

Exercise is not only good for your body, it also increases *human growth hormone* (HGH) production. HGH is a substance produced by the pituitary gland in the brain that helps our body retain calcium, reduce fat, stabilize sugar and insulin levels, boost immunity and more. Don't spend thousands of dollars on

HGH injections when your body can make it for free! Say goodbye to expensive HGH injections and prescriptions! Drink, eat, and exercise your way to a younger, stronger body.

The benefits of exercise are tremendous. It increases your oxygen intake and lowers blood glucose and also relieves stress and creates endorphins, the "feel good" chemicals in your brain. In the arthritis section we explained how exercise makes your bones and joints stronger, now we'll explain how it makes the anti-aging human growth hormone.

The fact that exercise acts as a major stimulus for the natural secretion of human growth hormone is well-known. HGH injections are very expensive and, in terms of training, research has shown that to achieve an elevation of human growth hormone above baseline, you need to spend at least 10 minutes exercising at above "lactate threshold" intensity. A lactate threshold is the level at which your body has insufficient oxygen to convert glucose to carbon dioxide and instead converts it to lactic acid. Any form of high-intensity energy such as sprinting, cycle sprints, tennis, etc., will do this. This results in the biggest volume of HGH secreted in response to a single exercise bout with levels of the hormone declining gradually over a period of an hour. It is also known that multiple daily sessions can give rise to optimal human growth hormone secretion over a 24-hour period.

One study investigated the effects of three exercise sessions a day with either half hour or three-hour recovery periods between. The study found that the longer recovery periods led to the greatest volume of 24-hour human growth hormone secretion. Another showed an even larger (HGH) peak in response to sprints on an exercise bike.

This means that exercise above lactate threshold induces the secretion of human growth hormone, promoting the use of fat as fuel. This in turn spares muscle carbohydrate, keeps body fat down and muscle mass high, and enhances adaptation to specific exercise stimuli. The benefits are clear, but simply switching to high-intensity work for the whole year is not the answer. The best way to get and maintain a lean body that produces good levels of HGH is to start en exercise routine that incorporates short bursts of intense exercise into a balanced routine of moderate cardio and weight lifting.

Important HGH Facts to Remember

Dehydration reduces HGH production.
Glutamine will increase HGH production.
Arginine, a component of protein, increases HGH production.
HGH production requires sleep; most HGH is produced one hour after falling asleep.

A suggested exercise and dietary strategy for optimizing human growth hormone secretion is as follows:

Follow an exercise program of three sessions per week each involving at least 10 minutes of work above lactate threshold or a number of sprints, with a 1 to 3 work-rest ratio.

Before exercising — no fat or carbohydrates for 60 minutes before; 2 grams glutamine 60 to 90 minutes before.

What is Glutamine?

Glutamine is an amino acid that is stored mostly in the muscles and plays a major role in helping our bodies purge ammonia, regulate digestion and aids brain function. Our bodies are capable of producing moderate levels of glutamine, but if you exercise regularly and/or do not have a diet rich in natural, unprocessed foods, a supplement is necessary.

During exercise drink plenty of plain water (i.e. 200 milliliters every 10 to 15 minutes if training in temperatures 65 F to 70 F.

After exercise, avoid sugar for two hours post exercise but take 25 grams protein immediately afterward in the form of either a protein shake, protein bar, lean meat or eggs.

Dietary sources of *L-glutamine* include beef, chicken, fish, eggs, milk, dairy products, wheat, cabbage, beets, beans, spinach, and parsley. Small amounts of L–glutamine are also found in vegetable juices and fermented foods, such as miso.

Exercise above lactate threshold level means exercise that will leave you gasping for breath. If you are a person over 40, make sure your cardiovascular health is in optimum shape by consuming adequate amounts of copper through your diet (see Chapter 1. We also recommend visiting your heart specialist and undergoing a treadmill test.

Since regular gym exercise can become monotonous, we prefer playing sports as opposed to general exercise. This is why Dr. Schep chose to join a rugby club and why Nicole has incorporated long-distance speed walking into her gym routine. Some great high-intensity sports include: rowing, tennis, running, soccer.

Commercial secretagogues are available to stimulate human growth hormone production, but it is questionable if they would be of use without exercise and if you have elevated glucose levels.

Don't waste your time and money on expensive hyperbaric chamber sessions and human growth hormone injections! By taking advantage of the natural benefits of air and water and the ability to move your body you can add years to your life, feel amazing and look younger and leaner. What are you waiting for? Take a few deep breaths, have a nice cold glass of mountain spring water and lace up those tennis shoes!

Secretagogue

A secretagogue is a compound that releases human growth hormones (HGH). Recent medical research has shown that the pituitary cells in aging patients can be stimulated to produce almost or just as much HGH as a person in their 20s. This has prompted a movement for prescription secretagogues as well as over-the-counter secretagogues such as ProHgh and GHR15.

While only one prescription, GHRH, has been approved by the FDA, that prescription currently is more costly than HGH injections (a price tag of over $1,000 per month!). Natural, over-the-counter products (ProHgh and GHR15) have proven to be very effective and can cost up to 90 percent less than the prescription alternative. Natural and cheaper — can't beat that!

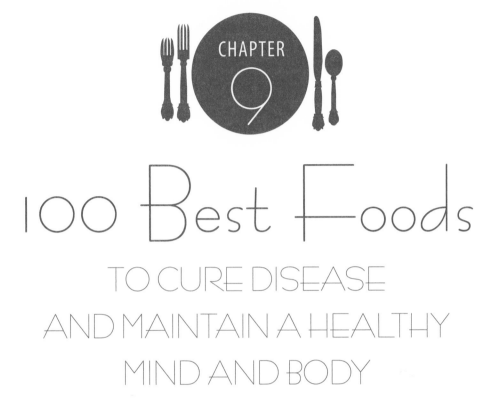

100 Best Foods

TO CURE DISEASE
AND MAINTAIN A HEALTHY
MIND AND BODY

Whenever possible, consume foods in their raw form. Raw, organic nuts hopefully will not have been irradiated (check for, and avoid foods with the symbol at right).

As cancer and heart disease currently are the top causes of death and suffering in the United States, we place an enormous importance on curing and fighting these diseases. Below is a list of 100 foods that help you fight these diseases and others, as well as keeping your body and mind healthy and young.

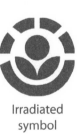

Irradiated symbol

The easiest way to start incorporating these foods as part of your everyday diet is to pick one or two items to start and build from there. For example, if you are having a salad for lunch, toss in some slivered almonds and sliced avocado. If you need a quick and easy snack, grab a handful of walnuts with dried acerola cherries. Sprinkle some bran in your cereal, add black beans to your salsa or pico de gayo, or dip your vegetables in hummus instead of dressing. Every day it will get easier and easier to eat healthier and, before you know it, you will feel and look great, not to mention you will be actively fighting cancer, heart disease, diabetes, arthritis, obesity and other serious diseases just by eating!

Each of the foods listed below has amazing health benefits. Following the list of foods, you will find a description of the benefits for each of the foods on our top 100 list. We recommend trying these foods raw first (when possible).

Acai berry, freeze-dried
Acerola cherries
Almonds
Apples
Apricots
Artichokes
Avocado
Bran
Barley
Bell peppers
Beans, dried
Beans, black
Beef and calf liver
Beef
Blackcurrants
Blueberries
Brazil nuts
Broccoli
Buckwheat
Bulgur wheat
Brussels sprouts
Cabbage, red
Cantaloupe
Carrots
Cashews
Celery
Cherries
Chia seed (salba)
Chickpeas
Cinnamon (spice)
Clams
Cloves (spice)
Cod
Cranberries

Cruciferous Vegetables
Cucumber
Collard greens
Dark chocolate
Dates
Eggs
Figs, dried or fresh
Flaxseed (chia preferred)
Garlic
Ginger
Grapefruit, ruby
Green tea (negative)
Halibut
Herring
Hemp seeds
Hemp seed oil
Hummus
Kale
Kidney beans
Kiwi fruit
Lentils
Maple syrup
Milk organic raw
Mushrooms
Mustard
Mustard greens
Nettle
Noni juice
Oats (avena sativa)
Oat bran
Olive oil
Oranges, especially
    blood oranges
Oregano

Oysters
Papaya
Parsley
Pecans
Pepper, black
Pinto beans
Plums, dried or prunes
Quinoa
Raspberries
Red palm oil
Rooibos tea
Rosemary
Red wine
Rice bran
Safflower oil (high-oleic)
Salmon, wild
Sardines
Sauerkraut
Scallops
Squash, winter
Strawberries
Seaweed
Sesame seed
Sunflower seeds
Sweet potatoes
Swiss chard
Tuna
Turmeric
Watercress
Watermelon
Wheat bran
Yogurt
Yucca

ACAI BERRY, FREEZE-DRIED

The acai berry, when in a freeze-dried form, has the highest Oxygen Radical Absorbance Capacity (ORAC) value of any known fruit, at 102,700 units per 100 grams. It also has the highest SOD ability (the ability to destroy superoxides) of any known fruit at 161,499 units per 100 grams. In the cancer section we pointed out that *superoxide dismutase* (SOD) was lacking in cancer cells, meaning that excessive superoxide caused the cells to go cancerous.

The downside to freeze-dried acai is that it can be very expensive, and acai powder that is not freeze-dried has not been found to have such high values. Nevertheless, it is a very healthful food for those that do not mind the high cost. The upside — a little freeze-dried acai berry goes a long way. One-half ounce (14 grams) supplies a whopping 14,553 ORAC units.

Acerola Cherry

Acerola cherries, also known as Barbados cherries, is one of the foods with the highest vitamin C content known to man. Vitamin C in adequate amounts is absolutely necessary for maximum ability of white blood cell to kill bacteria, viruses, and destroy cancer cells (see Chapter 7). Vitamin C also helps synthesize collagen for strong connective tissue and bones.

Although the fruit is not available in the USA unless you have an acerola cherry tree in your backyard (Hawaii or Florida), you can purchase Acerola cherry powder from health food outlets. One teaspoon a day of Acerola powder mixed with fruit juice or water can supply you with approximately 500 milligrams of vitamin C. Manufacturers also sell vitamin C powder (sold at health food stores) that consists of dried acerola, kiwi, goji, etc. The powder can be mixed with smoothies.

ORAC Value

The ORAC value is a measure of the foods ability to destroy free radicals, which are implicated in almost all diseases, especially cardiovascular disease and cancer.

Almonds

Aside from just being delicious, almonds are an excellent source of copper and manganese (good for fighting cancer and your cardiovascular health). It's also an excellent source of vitamin E and high in protein.

A 100-gram supply of almonds will supply 129 percent of your manganese and 70 percent of your copper daily requirement. Both in the Heart and Cancer sections we point out that superoxide dismutase(SOD), or the lack thereof, is a major factor in both diseases.

SOD contains copper and manganese and studies have shown that SOD in the body increases with copper supplementation. SOD prevents cells from becoming cancerous and prevents plaque from forming in the arteries. The 100 grams of almonds also supplies a good 129 percent of vitamin E, which helps the heart and makes your skin supple and smooth.

A good source of protein, a 100-gram supply of almonds contains 22 grams of protein. Eating raw almonds is the best way to go, as roasting almonds destroys the vitamin E content. Better yet — raw organic almonds. They are not irradiated.

Use almonds as a snack food instead of potato chips and candy bars. Almond butter can be put on celery and crackers and almond slices can be used in baking cookies, etc. Almond milk can be used for shakes or try plain almond milk mixed with a tablespoon of blackstrap molasses — two great foods in one!

Apples

Apples contain an exceptional anti-oxidant called quercetin. This anti-oxidant has the ability to protect against heart disease and cancer. The quercetin, however, is in the skin of the apple, so apple juice and apple-sauce lose some of their anti-oxidant power. Apple peel is now being used as an additive to increase the anti-oxidant level of some processed foods.

Apples also are a good source of fiber, which keeps the digestive tract healthy and prevents problems like diverticulitis (the intestines become unable to properly pass food on for elimination). The highest anti-oxidant content is in Fuji apples, then Red Delicious; Gala, and Golden Delicious being intermediate; and Cortland and Empire apples with the lowest amount. However, all apples contain good amounts of quercetin and other anti-oxidants in the skin and flesh.

The best apples of course are straight off the apple tree in your backyard (you can find great apples at farmers markets too). They normally have not been touched by pesticides or unnatural fertilizers. Second best are organic apples with supermarket apples coming in last.

Apricots

Apricots contain a huge and exceptionally diverse carotenoid content with one of the best-quality carotenoid mixtures. The carotenoids are beta-carotene, lycopene and almost 600 other carotenes. The carotenes protect against cancer, heart disease and macular degeneration by reducing the free-radical load in cells. Four apricots supply about 3,500 units of vitamin A and 4 grams of fiber.

Artichokes

Artichokes are of the thistle family and contain *silymarin* and *cynarin*. Silymarin is a compound that protects and heals the liver. Milk thistle extract also is being sold in capsule form as a source of *silymarin*. The liver detoxifying and protective properties of artichokes first came to the attention of researchers in 1966 (in a study that supported artichokes effects on liver regeneration in rats). A 1987 study that focused on the effects of rat liver cells subjected to harmful chemical agents, found *cynarin* and *caffeic acids* (both in artichokes) to have significant protective effects.

Avocados — Super Food

Here are just a few of the top things we love about the super food, avocados:

Avocados are a powerful source of lutein with other carotenoids which diminish cancer.

Avocados help absorb carotenoids in foods.

Avocados are rich in omega-9 oil and an anti-inflammatory, anti-cancer and anti-arthritis agent.

Avocados contain 271 micrograms of *lutein* and *zeathanthin* per three ounces. They are of particular benefit when added to a salad containing vegetables that are high in carotenes, such as kale and grated carrots. The oils in the avocado can increase the absorption of the carotenoids in the salad by as much as 10-fold during digestion. The omega-9 or oleic oil has a 1-1 ratio with the omega-6 oil, making the oil an anti-inflammatory, which is also of benefit for arthritis, heart disease and cancer.

There also are compounds in the oil from the avocado called "unsaponifables." These compounds are being marketed to stimulate cartilage cell production in the joints to combat arthritis.

Blueberries

Blueberries are a great source of body-protecting anti-oxidants and they even can improve your night vision! They have an ORAC value of 6,552 units per 100 grams.

The anti-oxidant phytonutrients called *anthocyanidins* (the blue-red pigments found in blueberries) neutralize free-radical damage to cells and tissues that can lead to cataracts, glaucoma, varicose veins, hemorrhoids, peptic ulcers, heart disease and cancer.

Anthocyanins improve the integrity of support structures in the veins and entire vascular system. Anthocyanins have been shown to enhance the effects of vitamin C, improve capillary integrity and stabilize collagen (body tissues are made from this protein). They work by preventing free-radical damage, inhibiting enzymes from cleaving the collagen matrix, and directly cross-linking with collagen fibers to form a more stable collagen matrix. This means that in addition to having a healthy heart, slim waistline and strong immune system, your skin will look younger and more radiant.

Bran (see also: wheat, rice and oat bran)

Sometimes it is difficult to consume only whole grains in our modern day diet. We are, however, able to get the benefit of the whole grains by eating bran (the coating removed from the grain kernels before it is processed).

Bran has a high insoluble fiber content. It can soak up many times its weight in water as it passes through the intestine. Because it causes the stool to become larger, the intestine is able to move the stool along more efficiently. This assists in removing toxic and putrid material from the intestine, thereby lowering the risk of colon cancer. (Colon cancer is fast becoming one of the major diseases Americans are fighting.)

It is suggested we consume about 15 to 30 grams of insoluble fiber each day. The breakfast cereal "All Bran®" contains about 25 grams of insoluble fiber per cup. Avocado, lentils, artichokes and most bean varieties, contain about 10 grams of fiber per cup. Of all brans, rice bran has the highest ORAC value (the strongest free radical destruction capability).

Barley

To avoid loss of nutrients and fiber in barley, do not use pearl barley. Like white rice and white flour, pearl barley has much of its valuable nutrients removed.

Of all grains, barley has the highest fiber content — 14 grams of fiber per cup. Fiber is essential for digestive tract health and the prevention of colon cancer. It is recommended that 15 to 25 grams of fiber be consumed daily.

In addition to high fiber, one cup of cooked barley has approximately 36 micrograms (50 percent of daily value) of selenium, an important cancer-prevention agent. It also has 100 percent of the daily manganese requirement. Manganese is a potent protector against cancer, by maintaining manganese superoxide dismutase (SOD) enzyme levels in the body. One cup (184 grams) of barley has 23 grams of protein.

The only downside of barley is it is a high calorie source of protein, so we recommend pairing one-half serving of barley with beans or peas to get a full serving of protein without sacrificing your daily calorie count.

Barley is unusual in the sense that it has the highest amount of *tocotrienols* in the whole grain, higher even than palm oil. Vitamin E can come in eight forms, namely four kinds of tocotrienols and four kinds of *tocopherols*.

Apart from palm oil, wheat and oats, which also contain some tocotrienol, all other plants only have vitamin E in the form of tocopherols. (Tocotrienols are considered more potent than tocopherols.) It is more holistic to have both in the diet, as each kind of vitamin E has slightly different anti-oxidative functions.

Barley contains 91 milligrams per 100 grams of tocotrienols, for a total combined value of 136 milligrams per 100 grams of all forms of vitamin E except *delta tocotrienol*. To get a complete serving with eight forms of vitamin E, you would have to combine palm oil with barley.

Enjoy barley in a lentil and barley soup or stew, adding a little of the super anti-oxidant turmeric and some soy sauce for a super-healthy complete protein meal. Amazingly, beer is considered good for bone health because the barley used to make beer supplies silicon.

Beans, Dried

Beans must be cooked in order to make the protein digestible, as uncooked beans contain protease-inhibiting enzymes that inhibit the digestion of proteins. Soaking the beans overnight in purified water can significantly reduce cooking time and reduce the protease inhibitor enzyme. Cooking destroys this enzyme. The trick is to cook the beans long enough (10 minutes) to destroy the lectin, but short enough not to destroy anthocyanins (anti-oxidants).

Beans are a powerful food containing a good amount of copper (cooked: 2 to 3 milligrams/kilograms), which is the prime anti-heart disease and cancer element. They also are an excellent source of fiber (6 to 9 grams of fiber per 100 grams/3.5 ounces), which is necessary for a healthy gut and to prevent colon cancer. A good source of manganese, the other anti-cancer element, a cupful of cooked beans will supply half of your daily requirement.

Dried beans have 8 to 10 percent protein content. Combined with any grain such as corn, wheat, barley or rice, they provide a complete protein (the same as in meat). (Beans are a great protein option for those following a vegetarian diet). One downfall with relying on beans and grains as your only protein intake — too many calories in order to get enough protein.

Beans have an excellent *molybdenum* content. Molybdenum is part of the *aldehyde oxidase* enzyme, which detoxifies the body of aldehyde and sulfite. Aldehyde results from alcohol consumption. Alcohol itself is not toxic. It is converted by the body into toxic aldehyde and then to harmless acetic acid. If levels of aldehyde become too high, it causes the toxic effects of excess alcohol consumption.

One cup of cooked beans will supply your daily requirement. Raw, uncooked beans have a very good ORAC value, around 8,000 units per 100 grams. Sadly, most of the anti-oxidants are destroyed by cooking. Brightly colored beans have the highest ORAC, such as black beans and the red varieties with garbanzo being the lowest. Nevertheless, kidney beans, after cooking, will have an ORAC value of only about 900 units per 100 grams. So stop cooking beans the moment they are soft and don't re-fry them.

Beans, Black

Raw, dry black beans, along with red beans, have the highest anti-oxidant score for bean varieties, or 8,040 ORAC units per 100 grams. Unfortunately, cooking lowers this score to an estimated value of around 900. The less the beans are cooked, the better; and soaking overnight can drastically cut down the cooking time and lower anti-protease enzyme (which creates gas). The anthocyanins work with manganese and copper (SOD) to provide anti-cancer activity. High in molybdenum (172 percent) raw black beans also contain 64 percent folate, 56 percent tryptophan and it has 15 grams of protein (30 percent), 20 percent copper and only 227 calories.

Beef and Calf Liver

Sadly, some of the most nutritious foods available are also the most neglected in the modern American diet. Liver is an amazing dietary tool. It is a powerful source of copper, which fights heart disease and cancer, contains *carnosine* (an anti-aging nutrient) and it supplies large amounts of vitamin B12.

Beef liver is criticized as being high in cholesterol, but in Chapter 1, on heart dis-

ease, we show that cholesterol has nothing to do with heart disease; it actually is due to a lack of anti-oxidants and copper. Beef liver has a food completeness score of 67 (highest is 100) and is complete in protein, vitamin A, thiamine, riboflavin, niacin, B6, folate, B12, pantothenic acid, selenium, copper, manganese, zinc, phosphorous and iron.

As with other meats, liver lacks fiber, but that easily can be corrected by eating it with a side dish of cruciferous vegetables, sautéed onions, or by "breading" it with a combination of finely chopped almonds and whole-grain bread crumbs.

Liver contains around 30 milligrams/kilogram of copper, which means eight ounces will provide you a whopping 6.8 milligrams of copper or 340 percent of your requirement. It also contains around 250 milligrams per 100 grams of *carnosine*. Carnosine is highly concentrated in the brain and may prevent aging of the brain (Alzheimer's). From eight ounces you also will get 565 milligrams *L-carnosine,* an anti-aging nutrient because it prevents glycation (see Chapter 2, dieting); and it lengthens "telomers" in cells. Telomers basically are the "expiration date" built into cells — the longer the better. L-Carnosine also has been found to have anti-cancer properties. You can get L-carnosine from regular meat and eggs.

Dr. Schep thought his local supermarket did not carry liver, as he could not find it anywhere in the meat section. A quick inquiry revealed that liver was not packaged like the other meats, but was sold in round white plastic containers, the same as cottage cheese containers, and it was dirt cheap! Amazing, especially because its nutritional value is more than 10 times that of muscle meat!

Beef

Beef is our No. 1 choice of animal protein. We rate beef above chicken and turkey because beef protein is 98 percent digestible as compared to the birds that are 95 percent digestible. Even a relatively small amount of undigested protein is not desirable moving through the bowel. A 3 percent advantage is very beneficial.

The only downside is that corn-fed beef has 30 percent more fat than grass-fed beef, but fat does not elevate blood glucose like carbohydrates do.

Beef also supplies:

L-Carnosine, a powerful anti-oxidant with anti-aging and anti-cancer properties.

Selenium, an anti-cancer ingredient.

A very high percentage of easily digestible protein.

The big difference between beef liver and plain beef (steak, rib cuts, roasts, etc.) is that plain beef is a poor source of the anti-heart disease component — copper (one milligram per kilogram or less). Eight ounces of beef contains the following daily requirements: 128 percent of high-quality protein, 94 percent of vitamin B12, 80 percent of the anti-cancer element selenium, 86 percent zinc and 50 percent of your iron needs.

Beets

Beets contain a colorful ingredient called *betacyanin* (an anti-cancer and powerful tumor-fighting agent). It is given as one of the reasons for the long and healthy lives of Russian centenarians as it is an ingredient of the traditional Russian soup called *borscht*.

In a study by Alexander Ferenczi [65], beet juice was used with some success to treat cancer in terminally ill patients. It also was found to prevent cell mutations caused by common cancer-causing substances (G.J. Kapadia [66]). Beets are an excellent source of folate (B vitamin), which also protects against heart disease, cancers, and birth defects.

Bell Peppers

Bell peppers have a mild taste and are easily added to salads, stir-fry, sandwiches and wraps, eaten alone or dipped in hummus or cream cheese. Not only do they taste good, they are a terrific source of vitamin C, with 3 ounces (100 grams) containing 316 percent of your daily requirement!

The vitamin A content of 3 ounces bell peppers is 114 percent of your daily requirement and it is in the form of various carotenes. One of the carotenes, lycopene, has been found to occur in much lower levels in the bodies of those with prostate cancer than those who do not have it. Another carotene is *beta-cryptoxanthin*. Smokers with higher levels of this carotene in their blood tended to have less lung cancer and emphysema than those with low levels.

As peppers are of the nightshade family (tomato, eggplant, potato, tobacco) these should be avoided by arthritis sufferers. There are compounds in these vegetables that promote inflammation, pain and stiffness in joints and even colon inflammation. If you do not have these problems, enjoy the benefits and the flavors of this amazing food.

Blackcurrants

Blackcurrants were banned in the United States for the past 100 years. They were accused of spreading fungus to lumber forests. However, blackcurrants are making a comeback and can be found in dried form in specialty stores. We are happy they are back because they are a potent source of vitamin C, the anti-infection vitamin. One cup (112 grams) of the currants contain 338 percent of the daily requirement of vitamin C. They have been found to contain even more anthocyanins than blueberries, and a study by B. L. Halverson[67] indicated they have greater anti-oxidant capacity than expected due to some unknown anti-oxidants present. Anthocyanins suppress cancer, heart disease and brain degeneration such as Alzheimer's.

Brazil Nuts

Brazil nuts have the highest known source of selenium of any nut. Selenium makes an enzyme in the body called *glutathione peroxidase*, which destroys *hydroxyl radicals*. Hydroxyl radicals can increase the formation of superoxide radicals, which some scientists have shown are in excessive amounts in cancer cells. If the level of superoxide can be lowered, the cancer cells revert to normal cells. Selenium also assists in the formation of the thyroid hormone in the thyroid gland.

An excellent source of copper, three-fourths cup of Brazil nuts will supply you with your daily requirement of this mineral, which is important for fighting cancer and heart disease.

Broccoli

One of the best vegetables in the cruciferous family, broccoli is a super cancer fighter. Raw is absolutely the best way to consume it, second best is lightly steamed. Microwaving destroys much of the nutrients. One cup of broccoli has: 123 milligrams of vitamin C (206 percent of your daily need), 155 mil-

ligrams of vitamin K (194 percent of your need) and 2,280 international units (IU) of vitamin A (46 percent of your daily needed amount). This one-cup serving only has 44 calories, an excellent food to limit the intake of damaging calories and to help lose weight.

Brussels Sprouts

Brussels sprouts are a standout vegetable in the cruciferous family. They are an excellent source of the anti-cancer *sulforaphane* and *glucosinolates*. We recommend steaming them very lightly so you don't destroy the enzyme that forms the sulforaphane and glucosinolates.

Studies showed that men who consumed 300 grams (about three-fourths of a pound) of cooked brussels sprouts daily for three weeks had 28 percent less DNA damage in their bodies. Brussels sprouts reduced precancerous lesions in the liver by 85 to 91 percent as opposed to red cabbage, which reduces them 19 to 50 percent. Brussels sprouts reduced precancerous lesions and polyps in the colon by about 41 to 52 percent. One cup (156 grams) of the sprouts provides 160 percent of your daily requirement for vitamin C, 18 percent manganese, and a relatively high 8 percent of your protein requirement.

Buckwheat Groats

Buckwheat is a gluten-free grain, a good source of copper (5 milligram/kilogram) and an excellent source of manganese. Three and one-half ounces will provide your full daily requirement. Copper and manganese form superoxide dismutase, which destroys harmful free radicals in the body that promote cancer and heart disease.

Raw buckwheat groats make an excellent cereal component rich in anti-cancer and anti-heart disease flavonoids such as *rutin* and *quercetin*. Rutin prevents platelets from clumping in the blood. Vitamin E enhances the effect of the flavonoids as the flavonoids protect the watery portion of the cells, whereas vitamin E protects the fatty part of the cells. The ORAC value is estimated to be 17,000 units per 100 grams or 3.5 ounces, so as little as one ounce will give you the recommended 5,000 units. ORAC, or oxygen radical absorbance capacity, is defined as the amount of anti-oxidants in 100 grams of food that has the same anti-oxidant capacity as *trolox*, a compound similar to vitamin E. The amount of trolox is measured in micromoles (17,000 micromoles of trolox is 4.25 grams. So 100 grams or 3.5 ounces of groats has the same anti-oxidant capability as 4.25 grams of trolox). Hereafter we will give ORAC values as units per 100 grams.

Buckwheat contains a high-quality protein with an amino acid score of 99 percent (100 is a perfect score). It also contains approximately 335 calories per 100 grams or 3.5 ounces, so the calorie load is low and the nutritional load is high. Another benefit — the carbohydrates in the buckwheat are digested slowly, avoiding the dumping of glucose into the blood. Raw buckwheat groats make an excellent cereal with raw milk, almond milk and some blackstrap molasses. It is also good for the gums.

Bulgur Wheat (Whole-Wheat Grain)

This is what regular, whole-wheat grain is called. It is one of the ingredients in tabbouleh (a finely chopped salad with tomatoes, parsley, mint, scallions and bulgur wheat). It contains *lignans,* which protect against colon and breast cancer. (Lignans destroy free radicals that make cells cancerous). Free radicals also damage the arteries causing cardiovascular problems. The carbohydrates in the grain are digested relatively slowly, thereby keeping blood sugar levels stable.

Bulgur wheat has a high fiber content, approximately 8 grams in one cup! This ensures healthy digestive action, preventing constipation, diverticulitis and colon cancer. It also is a good source of minerals: one cup (182 grams) will supply 1.5 milligrams or 0.75 percent of your daily copper requirement and 55 percent of your daily manganese requirement.

Cabbage, Red

Cabbage, as with all cruciferous vegetables, is a source of powerful cancer fighting substances. Unfortunately, cooking destroys the enzyme that releases these substances, so cabbage is best eaten raw or very lightly steamed. In addition, cabbage contains anti-oxidants such as polyphenols and anthocyanins, which are good for protecting cells against cancer, arteries against plaque and protecting the brain from Alzheimer's.

Red cabbage contains 197 milligrams per 100 grams polyphenols of which 28 milligrams are anthocyanins, while white cabbage contains about 45 milligrams polyphenols with only 0.01 milligram of anthocyanins. The vitamin C content is 6 to 8 times higher in red cabbage than white. If you like cabbage, then red cabbage should be your choice.

Using red cabbage to make sauerkraut will give you a superior food. Try shredding raw red cabbage into your salads or wraps for a crisp, tasty, disease-fighting meal.

Cantaloupe

Cantaloupe is a great source of vitamin A (anti-cancer, supports lungs, eyes) and vitamin C (supports the immune system).

Although cantaloupe is not as much of a powerhouse of nutrients as some other fruits, it nevertheless is a good and delicious way to get you daily requirement of vitamin A and vitamin C. You don't need to eat food just for its nutrition. Cantaloupe is a good example of eating something because it is delicious and at the same time enjoy some health benefits. One cup of cantaloupe contains 68 milligrams of vitamin C, or 113 percent of your daily requirement and 103 percent of your vitamin A contents as carotenes. Both vitamins A and C lessen the free-radical load in your body, a factor in heart disease and cancer.

Cantaloupe is a great way to incorporate raw foods into your diet as we should eat raw foods each and every day. The perfect ingredient for smoothies, it also softens and sweetens vegetable juices or purees.

Carrots

Carrots are an exceptional source of beta carotene (vitamin A). One cup of raw carrot contains 34,000 IU of vitamin A, or 686 percent of your daily requirement. Beta-carotene helps to protect vision, especially night vision, by forming the pigment *rhodopsin* in the retina.

In a study of 1,300 elderly persons in Massachusetts, those that had at least one serving of carrots or squash per day had a 60 percent reduction in risk of heart attack. Persons in the top 25 percent of beta carotene intake had a 300 percent less risk of cancer than persons in the lowest 25 percent. Carrots also contain a nutrient called *falacrinol*,

which was found in a study to suppress the formation of cancerous colon lesions.

One surprising finding is that smoking causes a vitamin A deficiency in the lungs leading to emphysema. Eating carrots daily can prevent emphysema (although stopping smoking along with consuming carrots is your best bet). Carrots are one of those vegetables that actually benefits from cooking. The heat from cooking releases the carotene from the fiber.

Cashews

Cashews are remarkable in the sense that they contain the highest level of copper of all nuts, ranging anywhere from about 28 to 39 milligrams per kilogram. This means that only two to three ounces of cashews can supply you with your entire daily requirement of copper, which is one of the most important nutrients in our diet and is a critical factor in both heart disease and cancer. Cashews contain 11 percent protein and the amino acid score of the protein is 100 percent — a perfect score!

Celery

Celery is a satisfying and easy snack and adds flavor and texture to soups, stews, casseroles, stuffing, and more. It also lowers blood pressure, contains high levels of anti-oxidants, enhances activity of white blood cells and stops growth of tumor cells.

A member of the carrot family, eating celery is a great way to incorporate raw foods into your daily diet, which should be done as often as possible. It is a good source of vitamin C and contains compounds called *phthalides*, which relax the muscles that surround your arteries and allow the blood to flow, thereby increasing circulation and lowering blood pressure.

Celery also contains anti-oxidants called *coumarins* that neutralize free radicals and enhance the activity of white blood cells and *acetylenics* that stop the growth of tumor cells.

Add chopped celery to your favorite tuna fish or chicken salad recipe; enjoy the delicious tradition of eating peanut butter on celery stalks (add a few raisins and you have "ants on a log," a fun treat for kids); add celery leaves to your salad greens; give your fresh carrot juice a unique taste dimension by adding some celery; or add celery leaves and sliced celery stalks to soups, stews, casseroles, and healthy stir-fry meals.

Cherries

Cherries contain *anthocyanins*, which are used by the body to produce essential amino acids. Antioxidants protect the cells of the body from the damaging, aging and disease-producing effects of oxygen, nitrogen and UV radiation. Anthocyanins are natural pain relievers, an anti-inflammatory and they inhibit the production of COX-2 enzymes (see Chapter 1, Arthritis section). Natural anti-inflammatories are believed to reduce the risk of many types of cancer.

Cherries also contain melatonin, another natural pain reliever and COX-2 inhibitor. Melatonin helps to regulate sleep cycles. Low levels of melatonin have been associated with heart disease and increased cancer rates in night workers. The human body naturally produces melatonin, but only in darkness. Constant artificial lighting, present in most homes and workplaces, reduces the amount of melatonin that the body produces. So, one of the health benefits of cherries to modern day man has to do with replac-

ing some of the melatonin that has been lost to artificial light, unhealthy work schedules and unnatural sleep patterns.

Cherries, like most fruits, contain vitamin C required for our immune system to fight infection and cancer. Cherries also contain fiber, which is important for a healthy digestive system. Diets high in fiber are believed to reduce the risk of colon and rectal cancers.

Fresh cherries are delicious, but not available year-round. Dried cherries are a great way to add pizzazz to cereals, baked goods, homemade trail mix or even as a standalone snack.

Chia Seeds (Salba) — Super Food

Chia seed is unusual in the sense that it, like flaxseed, is an excellent source of *alpha linolenic acid* (ALA), which the body converts into omega-3 fatty acids. Omega-3 fatty acids are missing in the our modern diets, and necessary to prevent inflammation in the joints and arteries. Four teaspoons of chia seed will provide you with 4.8 grams of ALA, sufficient to cure arthritis and even prevent it.

About 66 percent of the oil in Chia seed is ALA, compared to flaxseed, at about 56 percent. Chia has approximately 16 to 18 percent protein content — an amazing amount — almost as high as meat and higher than eggs. Also, the protein is a complete protein with a amino acid score of 115 (perfect score is 100). Chia is an extremely high source of fiber. One hundred grams of chia seeds has 38 grams of fiber, essential for a healthy digestive tract and to prevent diverticulitis and colon cancer.

The unique texture of mixed Chia seed is a feature of its high fiber content and water-binding capacity. Chia seed can be added to many foods, including: cereal, soup, salad, yogurt, smoothies and baked goods. You can also add chia seeds to buckwheat groats with chopped cashews, almond milk and blackstrap molasses to make a delicious (kiss your cardiologist and oncologist goodbye) breakfast cereal. There is some question about digestibility of the protein in chia, so it is important that the seed be thoroughly chewed or ground.

Chia seeds are an amazing little seed that contains, among other things:

Six times the calcium of milk.

Three times the anti-oxidant strength of blueberries.

Two times the potassium of bananas.

Three times more iron than spinach.

Eight times the omega-3 of salmon.

Two and a half times the protein of kidney beans.

As much fiber as bran.

Tradition has it that Chia was used as a super food by Aztecs and Indians of the Southwest, giving warriors strength, and allowing Indians to cross deserts and long distances by eating only a few spoonfuls of seed a day.

Chickpeas

Also known as garbanzo beans, these are an ingredient of hummus. Used in the human diet as long as 7,000 years ago, one cup (164 grams) of cooked chickpeas contains 164 percent of the daily requirement of molybdenum, a trace element, which makes enzymes that detoxify aldehydes and sulfites in the body. Aldehyde is a toxic metabolite of alcohol and we do not always know if the food we are eating contains sulfites, so it is important to consume things that neutralize

them. Chickpeas also have 85 percent of our daily requirement for manganese and 30 percent of our copper requirement, which are part of the SOD enzyme that prevents cells from becoming cancerous or makes them revert to normal if they are cancerous. They are also a good source of folate (71 percent) and fiber (50 percent).

A one-cup serving of chickpeas supplies 15 grams of protein (30 percent) and the protein is a complete protein. This serving size also contains only 268 calories, which means you would only take in 800 calories if you ate enough to get your protein requirement for the entire day.

Cinnamon (Spice)

Cinnamon has the third highest ORAC score of foods tested at 268,000 units per 100 grams. It has been found to lower blood glucose levels by up to 29 percent. It also has been found to prevent unwanted clumping of blood platelets, a factor in stroke. It does this by reducing levels of inflammatory *cytokines* such as *arachidonic acid* and *thromboxane A2*.

In the December 2003 issue of Diabetes Care[68], a placebo-controlled study evaluated 60 people with type 2 diabetes. The 30 men and 30 women ranging in age from 44 to 58 years were divided into six groups. Three groups were given one to three grams of cinnamon, the other groups none. After 40 days, all three groups who consumed cinnamon reduced their blood sugar levels by 18 to 29 percent and their triglycerides by 23 to 30 percent. No significant changes were seen in the groups who received the placebo. The researchers' conclusion: Including cinnamon in the diets of people with type 2 diabetes will reduce risk factors associated with diabetes and cardiovascular diseases.

Clams are a powerhouse of vitamin B12. One cup of clams (including their juice) will supply 1,870 percent of your vitamin B12 requirement. Vitamin B12 is needed for the formation of healthy red blood cells and, with iron, helps supply the body with oxygen.

The one-cup serving of clams contains 176 percent of your daily iron requirements, 40 percent of your daily copper, 57 percent of your daily manganese and 79 of your daily selenium requirement. All of these are minerals essential for the formation of anti-oxidant enzymes in the body that prevent atherosclerosis and cancer.

Cloves (Spice)

Ground clove powder has the highest total ORAC score of all foods tested, coming in at a whopping 315,000 units per 100 grams. Almost all disease has been shown to be in some way involved in excess free-radical activity in the body, especially cardiovascular disease and cancer. This means that a half teaspoon of clove powder will supply you with 3,500 ORAC units, right in the recommended dietary intake range of 3,000 to 5,000 units.

Cod

Along with wild salmon, cod is a great source of omega-3 fatty acids. Omega-3 fatty acids not only cure or prevent arthritis, but many studies show that they have a pronounced affect on the brain too. Studies on the elderly showed that all cognitive functions were beneficially affected and significantly reduced mental decline over time. This is a result of the ability of omega-3 to reduce the harmful inflammatory processes that would otherwise occur in the brain (K. N. Green[69]). Another study showed that a form of Omega-3 was highly effective in reducing depression and associated conditions such as sadness, pessimism, inability to work, sleep disturbances and diminished sex drive (M. Peet[70]). Another study showed that there was a lower incidence of asthma in children when the intake of omega-3 increased (T. Nagakura[71]). This is despite the fact that the children received less than 100 milligrams of omega-3 acids.

To get the most benefit out of cod (or salmon), you must pay special attention to the method of preparation. If the fish is fried in oil, it is subjected to very high temperatures, which drastically increases the free-radical content of the fish. The heat decomposes the protein into *polyaromatic hydrocarbons*, which generate free radicals in the body. Numerous studies have shown that the frying of fish does not result in the benefits mentioned here. The fish should be boiled, steamed or baked. Better yet — eat it raw as sushi or sashimi.

Cod is 23 percent protein, has zero carbohydrates, and the amino-acid score is an amazing 148 with 100 being complete. It also is an excellent source of selenium.

Try baked cod with fresh lemon juice and a side of steamed fresh vegetables and a nice glass of wine for dinner. Make extra and add a cod fillet to the top of a fresh green salad for a quick healthy lunch.

Cranberries

Cranberries have a rather long list of benefits including, but not limited to:

Lessening urinary tract and kidney infections.

Killing or neutralizing viruses in the

body (such as yeast infections).

Preventing formation of kidney stones.

Contains polyphenols that protect arteries against plaque.

Contains a compound toxic to cancer cell lines.

Increasing the death of breast cancer cells.

Cranberry juice excessively sweetened with corn syrup or sugar can cancel the benefits of the cranberries. Try an organic brand or a "zero sugar added" variety.

Collard Greens

Collard greens are given special mention here as they have been shown in the laboratory to stop the proliferation of breast cancer cells. Like all cruciferous vegetables, they have potent anti-cancer *organosulfur* substances in them that prevent and cure cancer.

Collard greens are unusually nutritious. One cup (190 grams) provides these daily requirements: 980 percent of vitamin K, 120 percent of vitamin A, 54 percent of manganese, 44 percent of folates and 5 grams of fiber.

Cucumbers

Cucumbers provide silica, which is good for joints, skin and arthritis; benefits your connective tissues (makes body stronger); and is a great source of vitamin C and molybdenum. Silica, in silica–rich plants, is a necessary component of connective tissues, which includes muscles, tendons, ligaments, cartilage and bone. Cucumber juice often is recommended as a source of silica to improve complexion of the skin. Cucumbers are also applied directly to the skin for various types of skin problems, including swelling under the eyes and sunburn. Two of the

compounds in cucumbers, ascorbic acid and caffeic acid, prevent water retention, which may explain why cucumbers applied topically are often helpful for swollen eyes, burns and dermatitis.

Eating cucumbers is a great way to get those ever-important raw foods. Purchase organic cucumbers, otherwise you might get cucumbers coated with wax (the wax is sometimes applied to reduce spoilage). The skin of the cucumber should be eaten as it contains fiber and nutrients. If you purchase pickles, select a brand that has no added sugar, corn syrup, polysorbate, (made from ethylene oxide) or artificial yellow No. 5 dye. Check those labels! Beer, made from silica–rich barley is also a good source of silica (T.R. Casey[72])!

Cruciferous Vegetables

Cabbage, broccoli, Brussels sprouts, cauliflower, collard greens , water cress, radishes, turnips, kohlrabi, mustard greens and horseradish all are examples of cruciferous vegetables (a more complete list can be found in Chapter 4, Why Raw is Better).

Cruciferous vegetables, namely those of the cabbage family, are well-known for containing substances like *indoles and sulforaphanes,* which have good cancer-fighting ability. However, in order to do this, the vegetables need to be crushed or macerated such as in chewing or the making of cole slaw. This allows the enzymes in the vegetables to come in contact with bound cancer-fighting substances and to release them to make them available to the body. The problem is vegetables, like cabbage, Brussels sprouts and broccoli, are usually cooked. Cooking destroys the enzymes that release the cancer-fighting substances.

Water cress is an ideal cruciferous food as it is always eaten raw and tastes great in Asian-inspired dishes as well as a salad topper.

In addition, 2.5 ounces of raw broccoli contains about 3,000 IU of vitamin A and a good 93 milligrams of vitamin C. It is rated as an excellent source of vitamin C, vitamin K, vitamin A, folate and fiber.

Dark Chocolate — Super Food

Chocolate lover? You are in luck. That chocolate bar actually can save your life!

Dark chocolate and cocoa are derived from a bean and it is a super food, remarkable for its very high copper content. Cocoa powder is reported to have anywhere from 27 to 50 milligrams of copper per kilogram.

The problem with chocolate is that usually it is combined with large amounts of white sugar, which has no copper in it. For example, if bitter chocolate with 30 milligrams per kilogram of copper mixes with three times its weight in sugar (25 percent chocolate content) the copper content drops to 7.5 milligrams per kilogram. It still has a good copper content, but its calorie count jumped dramatically. Highly processed chocolate should be avoided — it contains way too many added sugars, hydrogenated oils and other unhealthy toxins.

Now, the good news. Along with being a cancer-fighting champion due to its high copper content, dark chocolate and dark bitter chocolate contain *theobromine*, a stimulant that causes feelings of well-being. Dark bitter chocolate also has a very high ORAC value; values from 40,000 to 80,000 units per 100 grams are reported.

A half ounce of bitter unprocessed chocolate could supply you with an ORAC value of 5,000. However, cooking or excessive heating may greatly reduce the ORAC value. As a result, with both the copper and the ORAC value, chocolate has a double whammy anti-cancer and heart disease positive effect. The high level of anti-oxidants and the copper boosts superoxide dismutase (SOD), which destroys heart disease and cancer-causing free radicals.

Dates

Joe Vinson, in the Journal of the American College of Nutrition, 2005[73] had the following to say about figs and dates: "Dates have the highest concentration of polyphenols, (vitamin C-like anti-oxidants) among the dried fruits. The process to produce dried fruit significantly decreases phenols in the fruits on a dry weight basis. Compared with vitamins C and E, dried fruits have superior quality antioxidants." Conclusion: Dried fruits are a convenient and superior source of some nutrients, but in the American diet amount to less than 1 percent of total fruit consumed. The findings suggest that dried fruits should be a greater part of our diet as they are dense in phenol anti-oxidants and nutrients, most notably fiber.

Dates make a fantastic sweetener for your raw egg and raw milk high-protein shake.

Eggs

Eggs are a complete protein and have been awarded a protein digestibility corrected amino acid score (PDCAAS) of 1.0, which is the highest possible score for protein in food. The fat in eggs is not directly converted into glucose in the body the way carbohydrates are, so they do not impact the blood sugar like high-carbohydrate foods.

The best eggs you can buy are organic omega-3 eggs. You get omega-3 eggs by including some flaxseed or spirulina in the diet of chickens. The chickens will convert the linolenic acid in these foods onto omega-3 fatty acids for you. Omega-3 stops arthritis and stroke.

Organic eggs are a bit more expensive, but the health benefits greatly outweigh the extra dollar or two; and they are an economical source of the highest quality protein, higher quality even than sirloin steak (but much cheaper). Instead of trying to fuel your body with sugar cereals or nutritionally empty, high-carbohydrate foods, fire it up for the day with an omelet, scrambled eggs or a hard-boiled egg.

Figs (Dried or Fresh)

Figs supply both carotenoids and polyphenols. Figs and dried plums have the best nutrient score among the varieties of dried fruits (J. Vinson[73]). The anti-oxidants in figs can enrich *lipoproteins* in plasma and protect them from subsequent oxidation.

In humans, figs also produce a significant increase in plasma anti-oxidant capacity for about four hours after consumption, even overcoming the oxidative stress of consuming high-fructose corn syrup in a carbonated soft drink.

Try adding dried figs to your homemade trail mix for an anti-oxidant and energy boost.

Flaxseed

While chia seed is preferred to flaxseed as a vegetarian source of omega-3 for the body, flaxseed also helps kidney function, reduces cholesterol and helps relieve inflammation in your muscles and joints. Flaxseed can be purchased in its seed form or in an oil form. Some concern has been expressed about cyanide in flaxseeds, but the consensus is that the exposure is minimal.

Fennel

Fennel is another food that can be eaten raw, the ideal form in which to eat foods. Fennel contains *anethole,* which has been found to shut down the signaling process between cells that generate molecules that trigger inflammation, one of the factors for boosting cancer.

Garlic (Organic)

Nutritionally, garlic has a completeness score of 60 (maximum score is 100) and raw garlic supplies adequate amounts of vitamin C, thiamine, vitamin B6, selenium, manganese, copper, phosporous and calcium.

The benefits of organic garlic are many, including:

Organosulfur compounds prevent platelet clumping of blood.

Lessens plaque and dissolves plaque in arteries.

Increases blood flow by relaxing arteries; reduces inflammation.

Has potent antibiotic capabilities.

Manganese and organosulfur compounds give it anti-cancer activity.

Cooking garlic with meat reduces the production of the cancer-causing chemicals that result from grilling meat using high temperatures. You can marinate meat (lamb, beef) by rubbing crushed garlic in it before barbecuing.

Chopping or crushing the garlic stimulates the process of releasing the organosulfur compounds by releasing the enzymes required for the conversion. Crushing the garlic cloves before cooking provides the most benefit.

The organosulfur compounds in their antibiotic capacity have been shown to be effective against colds, flu, stomach viruses, and yeast infections.

Fresh, unsprouted garlic is the preferred form to use.

Ginger

Ginger is an amazing food that has been found to suppress the inflammatory compounds formed in joints, thereby giving relief to joint pain and swelling. Some of ginger's other benefits:

Contains carminative (reduces gas and bloating).

Reduces motion sickness and seasickness.

Safe natural aid for reducing morning sickness.

Relieves joint pain.

Reduces formation and growth of colon tumors.

Kills ovarian cancer cells.

Fights skin infections.

Used traditionally to destroy parasites and worms.

In studies by E. Ernst[74], ginger was shown to be more effective than Dramamine in reducing motion sickness, including dizziness, nausea, vomiting and cold sweating. In two studies involving as many as 675 women, ginger was effective in relieving the severity of nausea and vomiting during pregnancy, and was found to be safe with absence of side effects. Anti-vomiting drugs can cause severe birth defects.

Compounds in ginger, called *gingerols*, were found to inhibit the growth of tumors in mice injected with human colon-cancer cells. J. M. Rhode[75] et al, found that a ginger extract containing 5 percent of gingerol killed ovarian cancer cells in a number of different ovarian cancer cell lines.

Ginger can be taken in the form of tea and as little as two, half-inch slices (two-thirds of an ounce) can provide anti-sickness and pain-relieving benefits, but higher amounts provided more relief. If you are a sushi eater, take advantage of the sliced fresh ginger that usually accompanies your favorite sushi roll.

A purchased tincture with a strength of one to five grams/milliliters is recommended at the dosage of two to five milliliters daily. Standardized extracts of ginger rhizome can also be used with the recommended dosage of two 250-milligram capsules taken 60 minutes prior to the expected onset of symptoms and then two capsules every four hours.

Goji Berries

Goji berries have been used in Tibet for at least 1,700 years. Tibetan medicine includes these berries in the treatment of kidney and liver problems. They also are used in Tibet to lower cholesterol and blood pressure, cleanse the blood, treatment of cervical cancer, and use in the treatment of eye problems, skin rashes, psoriasis, allergies, insomnia, chronic liver disease, diabetes and tuberculosis .The people of Tibet use it to increase longevity and for overall body strengthening.

Modern science has shown that this bright red berry not only contains extremely high levels of anti-oxidants, vitamins and minerals, but also contains many unique *phytochemicals*, *polysaccharides* and complex compounds that scientists are just beginning to understand. Goji berries contain the following complex compounds:

Betaine, which is used by the liver to produce *choline*, a compound that calms nervousness, enhances memory, promotes muscle growth, and protects against fatty liver disease.

Physalin, which is active against all major types of leukemia. It also has been used as a treatment for hepatitis B.

Solavetivone, a powerful anti-fungal and anti-bacterial compound.

Beta-sitosterol, an anti-inflammatory agent. It has been used to treat sexual impotence and prostate enlargement (also lowers cholesterol).

Cyperone, a *sesquiterpene* that benefits the heart and blood pressure.

Grapefruit, Ruby

Grapefruit contains lycopene, the highest of all carotenes with the ability to neutralize the superoxide free radical (an activated form of oxygen) that makes it a factor in lessening breast and prostate cancer. It also contains *narigine*, which induces DNA repair enzymes to do their work — preventing cells from becoming cancerous. Grapefruit also contains *limonoids*, in particular, *limonene*. These are potent anti-carcinogens that remain in the body for up to 24 hours, whereas the phenols in green tea and chocolate only remain for four to six hours. So, a grapefruit a day will give you continuous protection.

A favorite healthy breakfast of ours is one ruby grapefruit with one cup All Bran® cereal.

Guava

Common guava, the one with the pink flesh, is delicious and provides so many health benefits. It is a powerful source of vitamin C (200 milligrams per 100 grams). Some general guava facts include:

Guava has been associated with healing of wounds when applied externally.

Guava has general *haemostatic* properties and can be used for treating a bleeding nose, gums and minor internal hemorrhaging.

Guava helps the body in combating

free radicals produced during metabolism and aids in preventing age-related chronic diseases, such as Alzheimer's, cataracts and rheumatoid arthritis.

Guava is one of the richest sources of dietary fiber and, thus, is good for those suffering from constipation. It has high roughage content, no cholesterol, less digestible

Green Tea (Negative)

Even though this is a list of foods we want you to eat to improve your overall health and well-being, we thought this information is important enough to put here to grab your attention. We do NOT recommend consuming green or black tea! Green tea is marketed and pushed as a super food that will fight cancer and free radicals. While it does have some healthy benefits, they are minimal compared to the high level of fluoride, which is very harmful to the body (weakens bones and interferes with the thyroid gland). You don't believe tea is laced with fluoride? See A. Diaof[76], he found from 3.8 to 11 ppm of fluoride in tea. The allowable fluoride intake for a 150-pound person is 3.4 milligrams a day. As a great alternative, we recommend Rooibos Tea.

carbohydrates and it is good for those trying to lose weight.

Guava strengthens and tones up the digestive system and even disinfects the digestive tract.

Guavas can improve the texture of skin and help avoid skin problems. For this purpose, you can either eat it raw or make a wash for your skin with a decoction of its immature fruits and leaves.

Juice of raw and immature guavas or decoction of guava-leaves is known to bring relief for a cough and cold.

Researches have shown that guava is effective in preventing cancer and heart diseases in people.

The presence of vitamin C and other phytonutrients such as carotenoids, isoflavonoids and polyphenols in guava has led to it being an effective anti-oxidant.

Guava also has been found to be beneficial for people suffering from the following ailments:

Acidosis

Asthma

Bacterial infections

Catarrh

Congestion of the lungs

Convulsions

Epilepsy

High blood pressure

Obesity

Oral ulcers

Poor circulation

Prolonged menstruation

Scurvy

Swollen gums

Toothache

In Chapter 7, you will learn the true way the body conquers infection using vitamin C; not vaccines and antibiotics. Sadly, ripe guavas may be difficult to get unless you live in Florida, Southern California or Hawaii. Most supermarkets carry guava juice, but fresh guava may be harder to find. Be cautious — the juice purchased in most supermarkets has little or no health benefit as it is high in sugar, high-fructose corn syrup and has been pasteurized. However, if you get the opportunity to buy raw guava, do it!

Halibut (Wild)

Halibut is an excellent food that is an excellent source of protein and the anti-cancer compound selenium. It is also an excellent source of the anti-arthritis and anti-heart disease omega-3 fatty acids. Frozen halibut is available throughout the year in most supermarkets and if you are fortunate enough to live in a city with a fresh fish market, you can get it fresh most anytime.

Halibut has 26 percent protein of very high quality (the completeness score is 148, perfect is 100). It is a complete source of niacin, B6, B12, selenium, potassium, phosphorous and magnesium. About five ounces (150 grams) of halibut will give you 38 grams of protein (70 percent), 100 percent of selenium and 830 milligrams of omega-3 fatty acids.

A few words of caution: Each year, hundreds of tons of farm-raised halibut are being sold to U.S. markets. Farm raising generally occurs in Canada, Norway and Scotland. Farm-raised halibut (or salmon) has as much as 2.7 times higher body fat content than wild sources, as the fish are overfed to grow and the fish do not swim; they just float around all day and eat fish chow with pesticides in it. The good omega-3 fatty acids levels are lower in farmed fish than in wild fish and the inflammatory omega-6 fatty acids are higher. Antibiotics and pesticides have to be used in crowded fish pens and the fish have higher PCB levels.

Hemp Seeds — Super Food

According to writer Lynn Osborne[77], hemp seed is the most nutritionally complete food in the world. Like some other seeds, hempseed has all eight essential amino acids necessary for life. What is unique about hemp seed protein is that 65 percent of it is a globulin called *edistin*. That is the highest in the plant kingdom. A globulin is the name for a protein that occurs in the blood. The best way to ensure the body has enough amino acid material to make the globulins is to eat foods high in globulin proteins. Hemp-seed protein also includes quantities of albumin globulin, a protein readily available in a form quite similar to that found in blood plasma.

Eating hemp seeds gives the body all the essential amino acids required to maintain health, and provides the necessary kinds and amounts of amino acids the body needs to make human serum albumin and serum globulins like the immune-enhancing gamma globulins.

Eating hemp seeds could aid, if not heal, people suffering from immune-deficiency diseases. This conclusion is supported by the fact that hemp seed was used to treat nutritional deficiencies brought on by tuberculosis, a severe nutrition-blocking disease that causes the body to waste away. (Czechoslovakia Tubercular Nutritional Study, 1955.)

Antibodies are globulin proteins programmed to destroy antigens (any substance eliciting a response from lymphocytes: bacteria, viruses, toxins, living and dead tissue, cancer cells, internal debris, etc.). Circulating in blood plasma like mines floating in a harbor, antibodies await contact with the enemy, then initiate a cascade of corrosive enzymes that bore holes in the antigen surface causing it to break apart.

One hundred grams of hemp seed contains 24 grams of protein and 60 percent copper, 150 percent magnesium and 100 percent iron of the daily requirement.

Hemp Seed Oil

Hemp seed oil, as sold in health food stores, is grown from a variety of hemp that has very low levels of psychoactive substance in the leaves and virtually none in the oil. It has a high vitamin E content (100 milligrams per 100 grams) as compared to olive oil (20 milligrams per 100 grams). The vitamin E is mostly gamma tocopherol, which complements the alpha tocopherol commonly found in vegetable oils. It is an excellent source of omega-3 and omega-9 oil.

Omega-3 and omega-9 oils: inhibit breast cancer, lessen inflammation in veins and arteries and inhibit heart disease.

Hempseed oil is ideal for use as a salad dressing.

Herring

Herring is very rich in omega-3 fatty acids. Five ounces of herring provides 2,055 milligrams and 238 percent of our daily vitamin D requirement, 100 percent of our vitamin B12 requirement, and 117 percent of our selenium requirement. That same five-ounce serving contains 20 grams of protein with a completeness score of 148.

Omega-3 fatty acids diminish cancer, heart disease and arthritis.

Vitamin D is a potent cancer preventer.

Vitamin B12 is anti-anemic.

Selenium diminishes cancer and supports the thyroid gland.

Herring is a great possibility for the recommendation that raw foods are the best. It can be consumed as pickled herring, but be cautious, most pickled herring in stores is loaded with sugar or corn syrup. Try to find some without, or try the recipe for pickled herring located in Chapter 10.

Hummus

Hummus is a highly nutritional food as it combines the nutrition of chickpeas (garbanzo beans) and tahini, which is made from sesame seeds. Because hummus is a combination of two healthy foods, it is quite complete in copper, manganese, phosphorous, magnesium, zinc, iron, folate, protein and fiber.

Hummus does not come with a calorie load because 3.5 ounces contains only 166 calories. This is an excellent food and tastes great atop whole-wheat crackers, in wraps, on sandwiches, or as a vegetable dip.

Kale — Super Food

If you are a cabbage consumer, you may consider replacing it with kale. For instance, cooked cabbage has about 2 to 3 percent of the daily vitamin A content in a three to four-ounce helping. And kale? No less than 272 percent per three ounces!

Four ounces of cooked kale has 272 percent of your vitamin A daily requirement, and 45 percent of your vitamin C requirement. Compare this to raw kale, which has 307 percent of your vitamin A requirement and 200 percent of your vitamin C requirement. This illustrates the argument in this book; whenever you can — eat raw!

Like all leafy vegetables, kale is high in the blood-clotting factor vitamin K. Kale also provides *glucosinolates*, potent cancer preventers. To get this benefit, kale should be chopped and eaten raw as cooking destroys the enzymes that release the glucosinolates.

Kale also has *kaempferol*, a flavonoid which has been shown to reduce ovarian cancer. Other carotenoids are *lutein* and *zeaxanthin,* which protect the eyes and lessen the chances of cataracts as well as promotes lung health.

Kidney Beans

Red kidney beans, up at the top with black beans, have the highest ORAC or antioxidant value for raw beans namely 8,500 units per 100 grams. Cooking the beans will lower the value to an estimated value of around 900. Soaking overnight can lessen the amount of cooking required, and hopefully leave more of the anthocyanins available. The amount of cooking time is a minimum of 10 minutes, see below.

A 177-gram cup of beans will supply 177 percent molybdenum, which detoxifies the body against aldehydes from alcohol and sulfites inadvertently ingested. It also contains 58 percent of your fiber requirement necessary for bowel health, 45 percent of your manganese requirement and 25 percent of your copper requirement. The serving has only 224 calories and it has 15 grams of protein (30 percent).

Anthocyanins, manganese and copper (in SOD) conspire to work against cancer in the body and the copper also works against cardiovascular disease.

Kiwi Fruit

Scientists have become interested in this fruit because of its ability to prevent DNA damage caused by oxygen in the nucleus of the cells. They have not found what in the kiwi fruit causes that, but that should not stop you from getting the benefit as DNA damage causes aging and, prevention thereof, will slow aging.

Kiwi fruit is a very good source of vitamin C. Three-and-one-half ounces of kiwi will provide 75 milligrams of vitamin C or 125 percent of your daily requirement. It also supplies fiber, vitamin E, vitamin K, folate, some manganese, copper, potassium and magnesium. It has a food completeness score of 55. Although it only has 1 percent protein, the protein is complete. It also has a low calorie count.

Lentils

Lentils are high in fiber, thus benefitting the digestive tract and an excellent source of molybdenum. In Asia, where molybdenum is deficient, higher rates of esophageal cancer are found. They also are an excellent source of folate and the potent anti-cancer minerals, copper and manganese.

Very easy to prepare compared to most beans, lentils have excellent nutrition. One cup of lentils supplies:

15 grams of fiber (15 to 30 grams a day recommended).

150 micrograms of molybdenum, (1,985 of daily value).

358 micrograms of folate (90 percent of daily value).

1 milligram of manganese (49 percent of daily value).

0.5 milligrams of copper (25 percent of daily value).

Mangoes — Super Food

Mangoes contain a generous amount of vitamin A. One cup contains 184 percent of the requirement of vitamin A as carotenes. But the amazing benefits do not end there. In 2002, Dr. Susan Percival[79] found the water-soluble portion of mangoes to have 10 times greater ability to prevent cancer cell formation than its carotenes, so its cancer-fighting ability cannot be judged by its carotene content alone. The water-soluble portion contains flavonoids and vitamin C. They have 76 percent of our vitamin C daily requirement and the flavonoids boost the activity of the vitamin C.

Mangoes showed the highest reduction of risk for bladder cancer (60 percent), which is the highest found in any fruit or vegetable. A true super-fruit with benefits,

including: tremendous cancer fighting capability, helps digest protein, is an invitro antiviral and a good source of vitamin C and flavonoids.

Mango has meat tenderizing enzymes in it, thereby making it great for chutney (only in its raw form). An additional excuse for raising it to super-fruit status is that the juice has been shown to destroy viruses invitro (in an outside environment such as a test tube).

The best thing you can do for yourself and your family is to make sure you always have mangoes around the house.

Maple Syrup (Grade B, Dark)

Maple syrup, particularly B grade, dark maple syrup, is a delicious, nutritious natural alternative to sugar and artificial sweeteners. Listed here are some of the great benefits of maple syrup:

Natural and nutritive sweetener.

Excellent source of manganese, an anti-cancer mineral.

Supplies a good amount of zinc, needed for the immune system.

The B grade or dark maple syrup (usually sold in health food stores) may be more concentrated (darker in color) and therefore may have a higher nutrient content.

Milk (Raw, Organic)

Milk is an excellent food, but only if it is raw unpasteurized and not homogenized. Unfortunately, the pasteurization process destroys all the enzymes and vitamin C in milk.

Raw milk contains *lipase* which digests fat; bacteria that makes *lactase,* which digests the lactose; and *phospatase,* which helps absorb calcium. All of these enzymes are destroyed during pasteurization.

In just one cup, raw milk provides 40 percent of your daily iodine requirement. Iodine is an important element that supports the thyroid. Vitamin D in the milk is a potent anti-cancer substance and, if cows are fed red clover, the milk will contain omega-3 fatty acids, which suppresses breast cancer.

Raw milk is a whole food supplying:
Protein
Good fat
Lactose
Iodine
Calcium
Vitamin D
Vitamin B12
Vitamin A
Omega-3 fatty acids (if cows are fed red clover)

Mushrooms

Activate your immune system to fight cancer with these little babies that pack a huge amount of nutrients into a little package. Mushrooms contain powerful nutrients and have been shown to contain *lentinan*, a starchy material, which, when administered to humans with gastric cancer, caused white blood cells and T cells to destroy cancer cells. They also contain *L- Ergothioneine*, a powerful anti-oxidant that destroys reactive oxygen species (ROS) that protects the liver and lessens cataract development in the eyes. (Patients with more cataracts had less L- ergothioneine in their eyes.) L- ergothioneine increases *Mn SOD* activity, the lack thereof that is the cause of cancer.

Shiitake mushrooms are the highest in L-ergothioneine and contain three times more than portobello mushrooms. They traditionally are an ingredient of miso soup.

We suggest sautéing mushrooms with onions and garlic. Serve as a side dish or as a topping for meat dishes. To give your vegetable stock an extra depth, add dried shiitake mushrooms. We also like to add mushrooms to our spaghetti sauce.

Mustard Plant

Mustard is made from the seeds of the mustard plant, which is part of the Brassica family (think cabbage) and therefore contains the same potent anti-cancer *isothiocyanates* that other Brassica family members do.

Believe it or not, a loaded hot dog with sauerkraut and mustard actually may be a healthy, disease-fighting food (on a whole-wheat bun of course!).

When shopping for mustard, make sure to avoid mustard that is loaded with sugar and yellow No. 5 dye. French's® Classic Mustard contains the super anti-oxidant turmeric (very smart) as it colors the mustard yellow without yellow No. 5 dye. We suggest you make your own (see Chapter 10: Recipes) and put in as much turmeric as you can tolerate.

Mustard Greens

Mustard greens are packed with nutrients. They provide excellent amounts of nine vitamins, seven minerals, dietary fiber and protein. Being a member of the Brassica family along with broccoli, cabbage and Brussels sprouts, they also feature the health-promoting anti-cancer *phytonutrients* known as *glucosinolates*.

One cup of mustard greens can supply 500 percent of your daily vitamin K requirement, 84 percent of vitamin A, 60 percent of vitamin C, 15 percent of vitamin E, and a holistic combination of anti-oxidants to provide protection against free-radical damage in the body. The same one-cup serving also will give you 12 percent of your daily fiber requirement.

Nettle (See Oats)

Noni Juice

In 1983, Dr. Schep was walking on the beach in Kona-Kailua, Hawaii where he noticed a bushy tree with very pretty green leaves. Hanging from the branches was a strange pear-like green fruit. Curious about his find, he picked the fruit and split it open. It had such a strong repulsive smell he thought it must be poisonous. After some research, he found that the fruit actually is not poisonous at all and has amazing health benefits.

Since that time, noni fruit has become a million-dollar product and the subject of hundreds of research papers. There are at least 10 papers, many of them by Ann Hirazumi[80], showing that noni juice has anti-cancer properties. There are at least six papers published that show noni juice is of benefit for preventing heart disease, and there are at least nine papers published showing an average of 30 percent lower oxidant free-radical damage to the body.

Research has shown that the human body requires trace amounts of *xeronine* to properly make some very vital proteins that are essential to the proper functioning of the body. It has been equated as an ingredient that signals to the cell how to function normally. There is very little *proxeronine* in our food due to the depletion of soil nutrients. Our livers convert proxeronine into xeronine. Proxeronine originally was discovered in pineapples (R. M. Heinicke[81]), but there

is 40 times more of it in noni juice.

Noni Juice is a potent source of proxeronine, promotes anti-cancer activity in the body, is rich with anti-oxidants and aids in preventing heart disease.

Noni juice must be purchased from a reliable manufacturer and not pasteurized or loaded with syrup and sweeteners.

Oats (Avena Sativa)

As we age, hormones in our body like testosterone and estrogen decrease. An anti-aging movement in the medical profession believes that we do not get lower levels of hormones because we age, but we age because of lower levels of hormones. We can get synthetic estrogens from our doctors, but these are not natural to the human body and have been linked with cancer. (They generally are made from horse urine — enough reason right there not to take them.) But fear not, there are healthy, natural ways we can increase our hormone levels.

Extracts of wild oats and nettles can safely help increase testosterone levels in the body (men and women both produce testosterone). The problem is that as we age, testosterone binds to a hormone called sex hormone-binding globulin (SHBG) and the testosterone becomes unavailable. There are natural substances that occur that prevent this. The most potent known lignans in this respect is the nettle root. In addition to inhibiting SHBG-binding, nettle root inhibits *aromatase*, which rescues the conversion of testosterone to estrogen.

In wild oats, significant amounts of anecdotal clinical observations, particularly with men in their 20s and 30s who had low testosterone levels for their age, have shown that supplementation with *Avena sativa* results in dramatically increased testosterone levels. The key to the effectiveness of wild oat supplements lies in the quality of the extract. Most extracts tested show little to no presence of the active *avenacosides*, which provide all of the potency. If you're going to use a supplement that contains wild oats, you'll want to make sure it comes from a supplier you trust.

Surprisingly, women are far more vulnerable to testosterone level changes as they have so much less to work with (even less if regularly using birth control pills). Because of this, even if a small amount of their available testosterone gets bound to SHBG, the results are profoundly disruptive causing symptoms such as:

Loss of energy.

Lethargy.

Loss of motivation.

Loss of interest in spouse and loss of libido.

Loss of fulfillment from sex.

Loss of muscle.

Significant increase in body fat. (The

prime reason women start to gain so much weight as they move into their 40s.)

Significant increase in the risk of breast cancer (bound SHBG is no longer available to lock up excessive estrogens).

Too much testosterone, however, can cause hirsutism (a condition of unwanted, male-pattern hair growth in women. Regular use of a women's testosterone-balancing formula can help to significantly reverse and/or prevent all of the above conditions.

SHBG binds not only to testosterone, but to all of the sex hormones including *estradiol* (one of the "active" estrogens found in both men and women).

Normally, this binding serves as a storage system for excess hormones, but in men there is an additional problem. SHBG also has an' affinity for prostate tissue. In effect, SHBG can serve to bind estrogen to cell membranes in the prostate. This causes an increase in PSA secretion — a prime factor in future prostate problems, including cancer.

The wild oats and nettles found in most men's testosterone-balancing formulas work together to reverse this binding process, thereby reducing the likelihood of prostate problems.

As we discussed earlier, saw palmetto has been proven to inhibit the *5-alpha-reductase* enzyme, the enzyme that causes testosterone to be converted into *dihydrotestosterone* (DHT), stimulating the growth of prostate tissue. The bottom line — regular use of saw palmetto in a regular routine helps:

Reduce enlargement of the prostate.

Tone the bladder.

Improve urinary flow and relieve strain.

Decrease urinary frequency (especially during the night by allowing the bladder to

Hirsutism

Hirsutism is a condition of unwanted, male-pattern hair growth in women. Decreased hormones is a problem of aging women. However, about 10 percent of younger women have an excess of testosterone causing hirsutism. Hirsutism is largely determined by your genetic makeup. But if you're a woman who has developed excessive amounts of coarse and pigmented hair on body areas where men typically grow hair — such as on your face, chest and back — you may have a condition called hirsutism.

A combination of self-care and medical therapies provides effective treatment for many women with hirsutism.

Spearmint tea, licorice extract and myo-inisitol have been found to reduce hirsutism naturally.

empty completely).

Reduce inflammation of the bladder and enlarged prostate.

The ingredients found in testosterone-balancing formulas such as saw palmetto, wild oats and nettle, work naturally in both men and women to enhance sexual desire, sensation and performance. The effect on human sexual appetite can be powerful. Both men and women can feel a boost in sexual desire (sometimes after only a few hours). Both men and women experience an increase in frequency of orgasms while taking quality extracts of wild oats and nettles, and many women experience a dramatic 68 percent increase in orgasms.

Oat Bran (Unrefined)

Oat bran is the material removed from the outer layer of the oat kernel when it is refined or turned into white flour. The kernel contains much of the nutrients in the bran. One cup of bran (3 ounces), contains 14 grams of fiber; that's 56 percent of our daily requirement. The fiber stimulates the bowel to work and keeps your bowel clean.

In Chapter 1 within the cancer section, we point out the effects of copper and manganese in the body and in the health of the cell. Cancer cells are low in copper and manganese SOD, and when these levels are corrected in the cell, the cell turns normal. With 265 percent of our daily manganese requirement, oat bran is an extremely good source of manganese to help form superoxide dismutase (SOD), which heals cancerous cells. Rich in SOD, it also protects the arteries against plaque and inflammation.

Brans are loaded with omega-6 fatty acids (approximately 8,000 milligrams per 100 grams) and almost no omega-3 fatty ac-

ids, so balance the bran with high omega-3 foods. The 100 grams of bran also contains 32 percent of the protein requirement, 19 percent of copper, 28 percent of iron and it only has about 231 calories.

Olive Oil

Olive oil has been used in food since ancient times in the Mediterranean. It contains polyphenols (like *oleuropein*) that inhibit both heart disease and cancer. The anti-oxidant-rich olive oil (also extra virgin olive oil and safflower oil) is loaded with omega-9 fatty acids. The darker the olive oil the more anti-oxidants.

The important anti-cancer and anti-heart disease effects of omega-3 fatty acids are highly promoted, but few people know that omega-9 fatty acids (oleic acid) are in the same standing (J.A. Menendez[82]).

In a very well-designed study, Menendez showed that both omega-3 and omega-9 fatty acids inhibit breast cancer cells, whereas omega-6 fatty acids (found in sunflower, grape seed and corn oil), stimulate the disease. Flax, hemp and canola oils all are rich in omega-3. Olive and safflower oil also place at the top of the list along with flaxseed and hemp oil.

The Menendez study is an extremely significant study because it shows that the omega-9 acids of olive and safflower oil are just as good as the famous omega-3 acids from flaxseed oil for cancer, arthritis, and heart disease prevention.

The anti-oxidants in olive oil prevent free-radical damage to veins and arteries and the omega-9 fatty acids lessen the inflammation in veins and arteries.

Use nutritional olive oil as a salad dressing and toss it with whole-grain pasta and grated fresh mozzarella cheese. When baking, replace the vegetable oil with olive oil and your heart will thank you.

Oranges (Especially Blood Oranges)

Did you know that just one orange contains 116 percent of our vitamin C requirement? Vitamin C is a critical component of our diet as the anti-infection vitamin.

Although oranges are not the most powerful sources of vitamin C on this list, the vitamin C it contains is of very high quality. The citrus *flavanones*, such as polyphenols and anthocyanins, support and enhance the effect of the vitamin C. Blood oranges are the most powerful source of the flavanones.

In a study of healthy subjects, those given 150 milligrams of vitamin C from real orange juice were compared to those who received 150 milligrams of vitamin C powder only. When the blood samples were exposed to hydrogen peroxide, no DNA damage occurred in the orange juice subjects but some did occur in the subjects on pure vitamin C. However, if the pure vitamin C amount is increased sufficiently, it will prevent DNA damage.

Oregano (Raw)

Fresh (raw) oregano is a powerful source of anti-oxidants and has an ORAC value of 14,000 units per 100 grams — five times higher than the average for apples. Dried oregano has an ORAC value of 200,000, which is the fourth highest score for foodstuffs tested. Pretty impressive!

Free radicals have been implicated in almost every disease, especially heart disease and cancer. One teaspoon of dried oregano will provide 2,000 ORAC units to the diet (3,000 to 5,000 is recommended daily).

Next time you enjoy a delicious slice of pizza or a big bowl of pasta, garnish it with some fresh oregano or sprinkle oregano powder liberally. Oregano also tastes great with healthy sautéed mushrooms and onions, adds major flavor to omelets and garlic bread and makes a great salad dressing when mixed with dark olive oil. (Boy, if that food list doesn't make you hungry we don't know what will!)

Oysters —Super Food

Oysters have a nutritional completeness score of 71, one of the highest scores for a single foodstuff. As one of the most potent sources of vitamin B12, a serving of 3.5 ounces (100 grams) of oysters contains 16 micrograms or 270 percent of your daily requirement.

The very same amount of oysters supplies 3 to 4 milligrams of copper, which is 150 to 200 percent of the daily requirement. Oysters reach super-food status because they also supply 672 milligrams of omega-3 fatty acids, putting your arthritis worries to sleep.

One hundred grams of oysters contains 57 micrograms of selenium (80 percent), 90 milligrams of zinc (600 percent) and 320 IU of vitamin D (80 percent).

Here's how all those amazing benefits affect our bodies:

Valuable as a source of copper (prevents and cures heart disease and cancer).

Potent source of zinc (supports the immune system and male fertility).

Good source of selenium (reduces cancer, and is cancer fighter).

Good source of vitamin D (anti-cancer vitamin).

Extremely potent source of vitamin

Farmed Oysters

Farmed oysters contain only half of the nutrients contained in wild oysters. One hundred grams of farmed oysters only contains 370 milligrams of omega-3 fatty acids versus the wild oysters with 670 milligrams. Farmed oysters also are more susceptible to pesticide and pollutant contamination. If you are unable to acquire wild oysters, purchase your farmed oysters from reliable shellfish growers. You'll still benefit from the nutritional factors.

Oysters are not a high source of mercury.

B12 (anti-anemic factor).

Excellent source of omega-3 (lack thereof causes arthritis).

Papaya

A small papaya weighing approximately 12 ounces will supply 190 milligrams of vitamin C, which is 313 percent of the daily requirement of this vitamin. As put forth in the infectious disease section in Chapter 7, vitamin C stimulates the white blood cells to be more active in fighting infection, and signals them to produce more hydrogen peroxide germ killer. Papaya also contains unique protein digestive enzymes *papain* and *chymopapain*. These enzymes help in the digestion of protein

Don't throw away the seeds, they are edible, highly nutritious and have a delightful peppery flavor. The 12 ounces of papaya supplies about 20 percent of your vitamin A requirement, consisting of *beta carotene, cryptoxanthin* and *lycopene*, among others.

Helpful in digesting protein, papaya makes a great salsa ingredient to serve with meat and fish dishes. Mix diced papaya, cilantro, jalapeno peppers, and ginger together to make a unique salsa for shrimp, scallops and halibut. It also makes a simple and sweet dessert.

Parsley

This vegetable is much more valuable than just decoration for foods. It has two major benefits. The first is volatile oils, which have been shown to inhibit tumor formation, particularly in the lungs. It also stimulates the production of *glutathione*, which then protects the body against free radicals and carcinogens. The beneficial flavonoids also help neutralize damaging free radicals.

Although one ounce of parsley might only contain 63 percent of vitamin C and 2,340 IU of vitamin A (48 percent), the hidden nutrients in parsley tell a much greater story.

Add parsley to your diet today. It's usually always available fresh and, to help you get started, we've provided an easy recipe.

Bring water to a boil. Pour in one cup bulgur, stir, cover and turn off heat. Let stand 20 to 25 minutes or until most of the liquid is absorbed and bulgur is fluffy and tender. Pour off any remaining liquid.

Using a small non-reactive bowl, prepare the dressing. Whisk together 1/3 cup lemon juice, one clove garlic, 1/2 teaspoon salt, 1/8 teaspoon pepper, and 1/3 cup olive oil. Taste and adjust seasonings.

In a large salad bowl, toss together 2 cups snipped parsley (no stems), 1 cup chopped green onions or cucumbers and 1/4 cup chopped mint. Add bulgur.

Pour dressing over salad and toss to combine. Taste and adjust seasonings as desired. Refrigerate.

Before serving, add a chopped tomato if desired.

Pecans

As far as nut species are concerned, pecans are the secret wonder. They have the highest ORAC score of nuts (anti-oxidant value), namely 17,940 units per 100 grams. Compare this to almonds with 4,454 units per 100 grams.

Like all nut species, they are a very good source of copper and manganese (parts of the SOD enzyme in our bodies which protect cells against cancer and arteries against plaque). A 100-gram serving of pecans supplies 1.3 milligrams (65 percent) of copper, 254 percent of your daily manganese requirement, 10 grams of protein and a whopping 10 grams of fiber!

The downside, of course, is 753 calories. But these calories come from oil and do not come with the destructive effects of carbohydrate calories (generates harmful blood glucose). Plus, the oil is predominately omega-9, which has the same anti-inflammatory effects as omega-3 acids. Although not the best source of vitamin E (8 percent in 100 grams) the vitamin E is of high quality, containing alpha, beta and gamma tocopherol.

Pecans are a tasty treat to snack on and simple to pack for work or school. They also make a great addition to baked goods and salads in addition to providing quite a nutritional punch.

Pepper, Black

Black pepper, while often overshadowed by salt, comes from a tropical vine (*Piper nigrum*) that fruits to peppercorns. When peppercorns are ground, they form pepper.

Black pepper has long been recognized to help prevent the formation of intestinal gas, a property likely due to its beneficial effect of stimulating hydrochloric acid production. Pepper stimulates the taste buds so that an alert is sent to the stomach to increase hydrochloric acid secretion, thereby improving digestion. Hydrochloric acid is necessary for the digestion of proteins and other food components in the stomach and is made from salt or chloride in foods. When the body's production of hydrochloric acid is insufficient, food may sit in the stomach for an extended period of time, leading to heartburn or indigestion. It can even pass into the intestines, where it can be used as a food source for unfriendly gut bacteria, producing gas, irritation, diarrhea or constipation.

Black pepper not only helps you derive the most benefit from your food, the outer layer of the peppercorn stimulates the breakdown of fat cells, keeping you slim while giving you energy to burn. In addition, black pepper promotes sweating and is diuretic, which also promotes urination.

The ORAC value of black pepper is 27,618 units per 3.5 ounces (100 grams) and also has antibacterial activity of benefit to the stomach

So, grab a peppercorn grinder, fill it with fresh peppercorns and shake away on your food for better health.

Pinto Beans

Pinto beans are the most popular beans in the United States, and for good reason.

Pinto beans, which are of Native American and Mexican origin, are low calorie, packed with nutrients and taste great. Similar to other beans, they supply 171 percent of your daily molybdenum, 74 percent of your daily folate, 58 percent of your daily fiber, 45 percent of your daily manganese and 25 percent of copper in a mere cup (170 grams). These amounts make them an amazing anti-cancer and anti-heart disease food. This serving size contains only 234 calories and has a whopping 15 grams (30 percent) of high-quality protein.

Plums (Dried or Prunes)

Manufacturers have been marketing prunes as dried plums to overcome the stigma of prunes being a laxative for elderly people. However, in Chapter 6, where we discuss bowel health, we point out the devastating effects that poor bowel health can have and the benefits of a clean and healthy bowel, no matter what your age.

Joe Vinson[77], states the following: "Figs and dried plums have the best nutrient score among the dried fruits. Compared with vitamins C and E, dried fruits have superior quality anti-oxidants, with figs and dried plums being the best. While dried fruits are a convenient and superior source of some nutrients, in the American diet they amount to less than 1 percent of total fruit consumed."

The findings suggest that dried fruits should be a greater part of the diet as they are dense in phenol anti-oxidants and nutrients, most notably fiber. The very dry plums found in oriental stores may have lost some of the polyphenols due to the severe drying process.

Quinoa

Quinoa, although used as a grain, is not really a grain but a relative of spinach and Swiss chard. It was a staple food in South America for thousands of years but cultivation stopped when the Spanish conquered the Incas.

In addition to the benefits of being a gluten-free food, quinoa also supplies copper and manganese (vital anti-oxidant nutrients), is a great source of fiber and a good food for complete protein.

A 100-gram serving of uncooked quinoa will supply 62 percent of your daily copper and 112 percent of your daily manganese requirement — the two most critical nutrients in our diet. This is because they are both part of the extremely important enzyme in the body, SOD, which prevents cells from going cancerous, prevents plaque build-up and makes healthy elastin tissue in the arteries. These nutrients are severely deficient in industrialized diets.

The same 100-gram portion produces 14 grams of protein with a quality score of 106 (100 being a perfect score). It also supplies 53 percent of your iron requirement, and 28 percent of your daily fiber needs.

Raspberries

Raspberries have anti-oxidants unique to them and possess almost 50 percent higher anti-oxidant activity than strawberries, three times more than kiwis and 10 times more than tomatoes. *Ellagitannins*, a family of compounds almost exclusive to the raspberry, are the largest contributor to their anti-oxidant capability and are reported to promote anti-cancer activity. Vitamin C contributes about 20 percent of the total anti-oxidant capacity, accounting for up to 30 milligrams in 3.5 ounces (100 grams) of fruit. Raspberries' anthocyanins, especially *cyanidin* and *pelargonidin glycosides*, make up another 25 percent.

Freezing and storing raspberries does

not significantly affect their anti-oxidant activity, but vitamin C content is cut in half by the freezing process.

Red Palm Oil — A True Super Food

Red palm oil is the biggest "secret" super food in the USA and should be the most used oil for food. Move over olive oil!

Can't wait to try it? Here's what red palm oil can do for you:

Prevent blindness and night blindness.

Prevent cancers.

Prevent arterial blockage and platelet aggregation.

Prevent skin damage and melanoma.

Prevent brain aging and Alzheimer's disease.

Lower blood pressure.

Enhance SOD activity (the anti-cancer enzyme).

Provide a rich source of beta tocotrienol (60 times more active then vitamin E).

Act as an effective anti-inflammatory (due to omega-9 fatty acids).

World palm oil production is second only to soybean oil, but recently soybean oil production has declined and palm oil has increased. Red palm oil is produced not from the coconut palm tree, but from the African oil palm tree. It is the most used oil in Asia and Malaysia.

Red palm oil is not just a super food but a super-duper food and following are the reasons why: It contains 15 times more vitamin A than carrots and 300 times more than tomatoes and it is the richest known plant source of vitamin A. The vitamin A derives from 20 different kinds of carotenes, each having its own special benefit in the body, including supporting the vision and the mucous membranes in the lungs and bowels, providing anti-cancer support, and even improves learning and mental ability.

One teaspoonful of red palm oil can provide a child with an entire day's supply of vitamin A. But wait, there's more! Red palm oil contains three times more omega-9 fatty acids (oleic acid) than omega-6 fatty acids making it an anti-inflammatory (arthritic, vascular and anti-cancer benefit). It contains no less than 800 milligrams per kilogram of vitamin E (compare to 500 milligrams per kilogram of vitamin E in sunflower seeds). And the vitamin E oil it contains is no ordinary vitamin E oil either. Eighty percent of the vitamin E oil is tocotrienols and 20 percent tocopherols.

Each of the eight forms of vitamin E has its own special function in the body. *Delta tocotrienol* is 50 times more potent than *alpha*

Red Palm Oil Production

About 35 percent of all this beautiful super food, palm oil, produced today is used to make biodiesel and burned. What a waste! It is being sold to people with the totally speculative claim that they will prevent global warming by producing carbon dioxide that can be recycled to grow new trees. So they are cutting down irreplaceable hardwood forests filled with monkeys and beautiful tropical birds just to plant palm trees to make a fuel, despite the facts: There is an almost unlimited supply of crude oil. (Biofuels can never replace crude oil as far as sheer volume required.) Also, the geological record (antarctic ice cores) shows that the earth has presently some of the lowest carbon dioxide levels in the history of the planet, and that chemically, carbon dioxide (only a trace amount of 0.04 percent in the atmosphere) has nothing to do with warming of the atmosphere [77, 78, 79].

tocotrienol, the most common form of vitamin E. About 10 percent of the vitamin E is in the form of delta tocotrienol. Research literature survey on tocotrienol finds that tocotrienol reverses blockage of the carotid artery and reverses platelet aggregation; prevents skin damage and melanoma; protects against brain aging such as Alzheimer's (C.K. Sen[80]), has activity against tumor production (W. Weng-Yew[81]); destroys excess free radicals from athletic activity; enhances SOD activity (the anti-cancer enzyme); is 40 to 60 times more powerful than alpha tocopherol in prevention of lipid peroxidation, which promotes cancer, and inhibits the growth of breast cancer cells (V.B. Wali[82]).

About 30 to 50 milligrams of tocotrienol per day is recommended. That's only one to two ounces of red palm oil. The World Health Organization (WHO) claims that the high saturated oil content in palm oil promotes cholesterol and atherosclerosis and that it should not be consumed. This has no scientific validity whatsoever, and Betty Kramer's reviews of the scientific work found the opposite to be true (*http://socwork.wisc.edu/new_web/?q=node/91*).

Your home should have a bottle of red palm oil in a dark closet or refrigerator, and tablespoonfuls should be added to smoothies, shakes, salads and beans and grains (after cooking of course). Dr. Schep personally keeps a bottle of it at work and takes a spoonful a day. "It tastes quite funny for a few days, but then, believe it or not, you get to like the taste."

Red Wine

Red wine contains flavonoids, and one of the important flavonoids is called resveratrol. Resveratrol is a bright red color and is an anti-oxidant much like the superoxide dismutase that the body makes from the mineral copper. Resveratrol prevents free-radical damage to artery walls.

While grape juice does contain the same protective flavonoids as red wine, the content is drastically less as the fermentation process for red wine allows thorough contact with the grape skins that contain the anti-oxidants. The mild alcohol content of red wine also has the benefit of relaxing the veins and arteries, thereby allowing more blood to flow and bringing more oxygen to the heart.

Red wine is considered to be "alcohol" in America and the consumption thereof is often discouraged, regulated, controlled and highly taxed. In actuality, it is a beverage that is healthful and almost medicinal, and has been around for more than 5,000 years. Before the days of trucks, trains and planes, it provided valuable anti-oxidant protection deep into the winter months to those who drank it when there were no fresh fruits or vegetables available to provide vitamin C in the diet.

Rice Bran (Unrefined)

Rice bran is the material that is removed from the outer layer of the rice when it is refined or turned into white rice. The kernel contains much of the nutrients in the bran. The unrefined rice bran is an extremely good source of fiber (stimulates the bowel to work and keep clean); a great source of manganese (forms superoxide dismutase (SOD) that heals cancerous cells); and it promotes SOD (protects arteries against

> # Tip
>
> Rice bran is more palatable, and the one study found rice fiber to be a somewhat greater colon stimulator than oat bran

plaque and inflammation).

Four ounces of bran (118 grams) contains 25 grams of fiber, which is our daily requirement. It also contains 838 percent of our daily manganese requirement. That is one powerful source of manganese!

Brans are loaded with inflammatory omega-6 fatty acids, around 8,000 milligrams per 100 grams and almost no omega-3 fatty acids, so balance the bran with high omega-3 foods. This amount of bran also contains 18 percent of the daily protein requirement, 30 percent of copper, 34 percent of iron and only 125 calories.

Rooibos Tea (AKA Red Tea, or African Red Tea)

Rooibos tea, or red tea, is a wonderful alternative to drinking regular and green tea, which are high in dangerous fluoride (see Seaweed section in this chapter for more details on *fluoride*). Some of the benefits of Rooibos tea include: Free of fluoride (one cup has only about 0.22 milligrams), caffeine and tannin, high in anti-oxidant content, protects against mutagenic and aging activity and it fights cancer

The Rooibos plant grows at high altitudes in the Cedarberg Mountains in South Africa with long days of intense sun exposure in the summer. This means that the plant has to protect itself against high levels of UV radiation. As a result, it is loaded with anti-oxidants.

Studies by Elizabeth Joubert[83] have shown that rooibos tea can destroy superoxide radicals. Therefore, rooibos is called a *superoxide dismutase mimetic*. Superoxide levels are found to be high in cancer cells, and when superoxide dismutase (SOD) levels are increased, superoxide levels are lowered,

and the cancer cells revert to normal.

The following data indicates that rooibos tea has 50 times higher superoxide dismutase mimetic strength than oolong tea and green tea.

This table is from Dr Nortier's Rooibos museum Web site: *http://www.dr-nortier.com/research.htm.*

Another recent study by Professor

TYPE OF TEA	SOD UNITS
Rooibos Tea	72,615
Oolong Tea	1,992
Green Tea	1,460

Jeanine Marnewick[84] using healthy volunteers, found that six cups a day of rooibos tea taken for three months elevated blood glutathione by 100 percent. Glutathione is the master anti-oxidant in the body. It is made by the body, especially the liver, and cannot be taken as a supplement because it is broken down in the gut. (It decreases with aging and smoking.) In many studies glutathione has been found to counteract heart disease, cancer and aging.

Rooibos tea contains very little tannin so normally it is boiled for about 10 minutes until it becomes a deep dark red color. This dramatically increases the amount of anti-oxidants in the brew. The ORAC value increased from 725 units per gram for steeped tea to 1,115 units per gram by boiling for 10 minutes (C. Fajardo-Lira[85]) and it still retains its sweet taste. Drink as is, or add a teaspoon of maple syrup (preferably dark). The boiled leaves actually are good for a second brew. See Rooibos Tea recipe in Chapter 10.

ROSEMARY

Some foods provide benefits gleaned from macronutrients such as protein and vitamins, but some have aromatherapy benefits (the aroma stimulates the brain to produce health effects). Rosemary is one of those foods and in addition to the wonderful smell, it also means good health.

Rosemary contains substances that are useful for stimulating the immune system, increasing circulation and improving digestion. It also contains anti-inflammatory compounds that reduce the severity of asthma attacks and it has been shown to increase the blood flow to the head and brain, improving concentration.

The next time you enhance the flavor of some special dish with rosemary, you will be making a healthy, and delicious, decision.

Safflower Oil (High-Oleic)

Safflower oil comes in two forms, high-oleic (omega-9), the most common and high linoleic (omega-6). High-oleic safflower oil normally is not considered to be a health food but bear with us and maybe we will change your mind.

Reported in a letter to the Annals of Oncology, J. A. Mendez[86] exposed breast cancer cells to omega-3, omega 6 and omega-9 acids. He found that these acids affected *oncogene* in the cancer cells (cancer cells have a high oncogene level). He also found that both omega-3 and omega-9 **lowered** oncogene levels (good) and omega-6 (ALA) **increased** oncogene levels (bad).

The most powerful lowering agent was the omega-3 fatty acid called DHA (58 percent), but GLA was 54 percent, oleic acid (omega-9) was 55 percent and ALA (omega-3) 45 percent and EPA (omega-3) 33 percent. Here it comes: Olive oil contains about 71 percent omega-9, but there is no higher omega-9-containing oil than high-oleic safflower oil — 74 percent.

Due to this study, it is important to minimize your intake of grape seed oil (73 percent omega-6), corn oil (58 percent omega-6), and sunflower oil (68 percent omega-6) as Menedez found that *omega-6 oil increased oncogene content* to 150 percent.

In addition, 3.5 ounces (100 grams) of safflower oil has a whopping 205 percent of your vitamin E needs!

Full Scientific Names for Acronyms

DHA: Docosahexaenoic acid (omega-3, fish oil).
GLA: Gamma-linolenic acid (omega-6, evening primrose oil, not to be confused with ALA).
ALA: Alpha-linoleic acid (omega-6, grape seed oil, corn oil).
EPA: Eicosapentaenoic acid (omega-3, fish oil).
LA: Linolenic acid (omega-3, flaxseed oil).
Oleic Acid: Omega-9 (safflower oil, olive oil).

Salmon, Wild — Super Food

In Alaska, fishermen do not allow salmon farming, meaning that only wild Alaskan salmon are harvested. As opposed to farmed salmon, this salmon has a high level of omega-3 fatty acids in the meat, which protects against joint inflammation, arthritis and coronary inflammation. The DHA it contains is a potent anti-cancer oil. The protein, being of a fish source, is of the best quality. It also has an amazing 40 to 60 percent protein content in the meat and the protein completeness score is an amazing 148, even higher than eggs (eggs rate 136).

We suggest you try to eat wild salmon at least once a week. Try it over salad or baked with lemon juice and fresh rosemary.

Sardines — Super Food

Sardines has been relegated to super food status because they are a powerful source of omega-3 (arthritis preventer), vitamin B12 (anti-anemic), vitamin D (cancer preventer), selenium (cancer and goiter preventer), and a good source of protein and vitamin E.

One cup of sardines (148 grams) contains 222 percent of the daily required B12 vitamin, 2,205 milligrams omega-3, 100 percent of your daily vitamin D and selenium, 73 percent of protein and, even though packed in oil, only 310 calories.

Stock up on cans of sardines and open a can of sardines instead of potato chips when you feel in need of a snack.

Sauerkraut and Kimchi — Super Food

Sauerkraut has profound anti-cancer benefits. During the fermentation process of raw cabbage (turning raw cabbage into sauerkraut), enzymes are released by a bug called *lactobacillus plantarum*. This "bug" not only produces anti-cancer phytochemicals, it also converts the *glucosinolates* in the cabbage to *isothiocyanates*, which kills cancer cells. The *isothiocyanates* also aid in digestion, as these dominating bacteria kill pathogenic (infection-causing) bacteria and stimulate the immune system to function better. Sauerkraut also helps break down the protein in the stomach.

When kimchi was given to chickens, it cured them of avian flu. Kimchi also cures upset stomach and constipation. However, you must be cautious of purchased kimchi.

Watch out for any that is loaded with chili.

Scallops

Scallops are an excellent source of protein without the associated calories. An 8-ounce serving will supply you with 90 percent of your daily needs for protein, 66 percent of your vitamin B12 requirement, and 30 percent of your omega-3 fatty acids. With only 302 calories, this high-quality protein is also a complete protein.

Eating scallops broiled or baked (not fried) may reduce risk of atrial fibrillation in the elderly, the most common type of heart arrhythmia. This is according to the July, 2004 issue of *Circulation*. In the 12-year study of 4,815 people 65 years of age and older, eating canned tuna or other broiled or baked fish one to four times a week correlated with increased blood levels of omega-3 fatty acids and a 28 percent lower risk of atrial fibrillation. Eating broiled or baked fish five times a week lowered risk even more, showing a drop in atrial fibrillation risk of 31 percent. Eating fried fish, however, provided no similar protection. Not only is fried fish typically made from lean fish like cod and Pollack that provide fewer omega-3 fatty acids, but frying results in the production of free-radical-laden fats and *polyaromatic amines* in the fish as well as the frying oil. In further research to determine if the omega-3 fats found in fish oil were responsible for fish's beneficial effects on the heart's electrical circuitry, Mozaffarian and colleagues from Harvard Medical School analyzed data on fish intake and electrocardiogram results from 5,096 adults, aged 65 or older, from 1989 to 1990.

Eating scallops or other broiled or baked fish at least once a week was associated with lower heart rate by 3.2 beats per minute and a 50 percent lower likelihood of prolonged ventricular repolarization (the period of time it takes the heart to recharge after it beats, so it can beat again), compared to those consuming fish less than once a month.

Seaweed

Seaweed is not just for wrapping sushi! This multi-talented plant has multiple names: kombu (kelp), dulse (sea parsley), wakame, arame and hiziki.

Studies have shown that in areas where seaweed is commonly consumed, there is a very low incidence of goiter. Although the recommended daily allowance (RDA) for iodine is only 0.15 milligrams per day, some studies have found that 10 times the amount (1 to 2 milligrams) is required to prevent goiter. The RDA amount appears to be just the absolute minimum to prevent serious disorders and may not be the optimum amount.

Seaweed is beneficial in many ways, including the following:

Anti-goitrogens (prevents goiter and low thyroid activity).

Supplies both iodine and tyrosine (a thryoid hormone and amino acid that the body uses to synthesize proteins).

Prevents and resolves breast, uterus and ovary lumps.

Less cancer has been found in animals with adequate iodine intake.

Lessens tendency to obesity.

Appears important for the immune system and prevents autoimmunity.

The medical community is warning against high iodine consumption causing an overactive thyroid, but if this happens, the remedy merely would be to cut back on io-dine intake. However, thyroid problems due to too much iodine may actually be due to a selenium deficiency as selenium works with iodine.

During Dr. Schep's research, he found that low thyroid, not high thyroid, is the major problem in the United States. Low thyroid results in lethargy (especially early in the morning), depression and cold hands and feet.

Goiter results in an enlarged thyroid which doctor's solve by surgically removing it, which can harm your vocal chords. Once your thyroid is removed, you must purchase and use a synthetic thyroid hormone for the rest of your life. Not the best solution by a long shot.

Low thyroid activity is caused by two factors: lack of iodine in the processed-food diet and disruption of the thyroid gland caused by fluoride poisoning. Fluoride chemically is similar to iodine but does not provide electrons as easily as iodine, as the electrons are more tightly bound.

Fluoride poisoning is largely caused by the consumption of regular tea, which contains large amounts (as much 4 milligrams) of fluoride per cup. A contributing factor is the fluoridation of our drinking water. In arid climates where water evaporation is high, this results in the fluoride content being elevated (brackish water).

Even though many people now purchase drinking water, fluoridated tap water is still used for cooking, making coffee, etc. One quart of water can supply you with 4 milligrams of fluoride. An intake of more than 1 milligram per day is considered toxic. Fluoride also weakens the bones and teeth.

Before the advent of synthetic drugs, doctors used fluoride to treat overactive thyroid. So if you have an underactive thyroid, you most certainly don't want fluoride. The thyroid hormone is necessary for the metabolism in the body, namely the burning of carbohydrates. And low thyroid hormone may be a contributing factor to obesity.

Iodine has also been shown to get rid of breast lumps and cysts and those of the uterus and ovaries. Clinically, 4 milligrams per day of iodine *removed* lumps in breasts within two months. One to two milligrams per day will *prevent* lumps and cysts. Iodine has shown to normalize abnormal cells.

Cancer cells are the most abnormal of all, so it is hardly surprising that increased rates of cancer have been found in animals with deficient iodine. The iodine content of seaweed can vary, even from day to day, but the following should be a rough guide.

Medicinally, five to 10 grams (one to two teaspoons) of seaweed per day is used. Dr. Sebastian Venturi says we do not even know yet what all the tremendous functions of iodine are in the body, but he is working to find out. He found iodine to be rapidly taken up in the body by the stomach lining, skin, salivary glands and even the thymus gland. The thymus gland has the important function of regulating the immune system of the body and preventing autoimmunity, which causes inflammation in the body. Arthritis and cancer are just some of the results of inflammation in the body. The thymus

glands shrinks as we age, and we all know that arthritis and cancer increases with age.

History indicates that dulse has been harvested and eaten in the British Isles for at least 600 years. Nova Scotia and the Pacific Northwest are also regions where dulse is regularly consumed. Kombu (kelp) is unusual in the sense that about 10 percent of its iodine content is in the form of *iodinated tyrosines*. These molecules can very easily be used by the thyroid to make thyroid hormone.

Dulse can be eaten dried, used in salads or soups and kelp can be used as a garnish.

Sesame Seeds

Sesame seeds are another excellent source of copper and manganese. They contain about 40 milligrams per kilogram of copper which means that less than two ounces will supply your entire daily requirement of copper and four ounces will supply your complete daily manganese requirement. Sesame seeds are unusual in that they have a very high *phytosterol* content, as much as 400 milligrams per 3.5 ounces (100 grams). Phytosterols enhance the immune response and in so doing decrease cancer risk.

Soybeans

Soy can be consumed cooked whole or in the form of tofu or soy flour. Soy is proba-

FOOD NAME	FOOD WEIGHT	IODINE CONTENT
Dulse or sea parsley	10 grams (1/3 ounce)	1.5 to 3 milligrams
Kelp or kombu	10 grams (1/3 ounce)	1 to 2 milligrams

bly the best vegetable form of protein as the carbohydrate load is so low. Soy flour has only 33 percent carbohydrates compared to buckwheat, which has 79 percent. The protein is of excellent quality and is a complete protein, scoring 118 for completeness.

Sunflower Seeds —Super Food

Sunflower seeds are a super food as they have the highest vitamin E content of common foods outside of red palm oil and wheat germ oil. The vitamin E basically is in the form of *alpha tocopherol* (95 percent) with a small amount of *beta tocopherol*, (about 5 percent).

It is best to get vitamin E from our foods instead of capsules as foods with vitamin E have both alpha and beta tocopherols, whereas vitamin E capsules only have alpha tocopherol. Capsules with complete tocopherols are available, although they are four to 10 times more expensive than regular vitamin E.

A half-cup serving of sunflower seeds contains 182 percent of our vitamin E requirement, 70 percent of both selenium and manganese and 62 percent of our daily copper requirement. All these work together to manage reactive oxygen in our body, another reason why food vitamin E is superior. This conspires to reduce inflammation in the body, responsible for such diseases as cancer, cardiovascular disease, Alzheimer's disease and arthritis.

Easy to purchase and fun to snack on, sunflower seeds have a lot more potential:

Protect your skin from ultraviolet light.

Prevent cell damage from free radicals.

Allow your cells to communicate effectively.

Help protect against prostate cancer and

Alzheimer's disease.

Vitamin E, if applied topically to the skin, prevents UV damage from the sun, prevents aging of the skin and increases the ability of the skin to retain moisture. It also can help prevent stretch marks during pregnancy. Make sure the skincare product you buy declares the weight of vitamin E contained in the product, otherwise it will only have a token amount. The higher the IU of vitamin E declared on the jar, the more E in the container.

Squash (Winter)

Winter squash is an excellent source of nutrition. One cup of winter squash will provide the equivalent of 146 percent of your daily vitamin A requirement, 30 percent of your daily vitamin C requirement, 25 percent of your daily required fiber, 15 percent or your daily omega-3 and 12 percent of your daily copper requirement.

The vitamin A prevents cancer, provides lung health and prevents emphysema. Vitamin C supports the immune system. Omega-3 suppresses inflammation and arthritis in the body. And copper is part of the SOD that protects cells against cancer and arteries against plaque.

Winter squash can be boiled soft and sprinkled with a small amount of brown sugar and liberal amounts of cinnamon, a powerful source of anti-oxidants.

Strawberries

Strawberries are a rich source of phenols such as anthocyanins (especially *anthocyanin ellagitannins*). These potent anti-oxidants are shown to prevent oxygen damage in all of the body's organ systems. The unique phenols in strawberries make them a heart-protective fruit, an anti-cancer fruit, and an anti-inflammatory fruit all rolled into one. The anti-inflammatory properties of phenols in this fruit lessens activity of the enzyme *cyclo-oxygenase* (COX) (see Chapter 1, Arthritis section) where over-activity has been shown to contribute to unwanted inflammation involved in rheumatoid and osteoarthritis, asthma, atherosclerosis and cancer. Unlike drugs that are COX-inhibitors, however, strawberries do not cause intestinal bleeding or liver and joint damage.

The *ellagitannin* actually has been associated with decreased rates of cancer death. In one study, strawberries topped a list of eight foods most linked to lower rates of cancer deaths among a group of over 1,000 elderly people. Those eating the most strawberries were three times less likely to develop cancer compared to those eating few or no strawberries.

A study by K. J. Meyers[87], published in the Journal of Agriculture and Food Chemistry, analyzed eight strawberry cultivars. All were able to significantly inhibit the proliferation of human liver cancer cells. Interestingly, no relationship was found between a cultivar's anti-oxidant content and its ability to inhibit cancer cell proliferation, which suggests that this beneficial effect of strawberries is caused by other actions of their many beneficial compounds.

Sweet Potatoes

Sweet potatoes are in the morning glory family and should not be confused with yams, which are in the *dioscorea* family. The bright yellow color of sweet potatoes means they are loaded with alpha carotene. Do not peel the potatoes — the skin contains three times as many anti-oxidants as the actual flesh of the potato. The darker the color, the more anti-oxidants.

The top 25 percent of carotene consumers have 200 percent lower cancer occurrences than the lowest 25 percent of carotene consumers. Sweet potatoes are unusual in that they contain root storage protein that has one-third as much anti-oxidant activity as *glutathione*, a powerful anti-oxidant in the body.

A 3.5-ounce serving of sweet potatoes contains the body's daily requirements: 340 percent vitamin A, 32 percent vitamin C, 33 percent manganese, 20 percent copper, and it only contains about 123 calories!

Sweet potatoes are best eaten as a side dish to a high-protein food, as it does not contain much protein (2 percent).

Swiss Chard

Swiss chard is a powerhouse of nutrition, containing high amounts of many nutrients. Six ounces of Swiss chard supplies you with the following daily requirements: 716 percent vitamin K, 110 percent vitamin A, 53 percent vitamin C, 30 percent manganese, 25 percent iron and 17 percent of your vitamin E requirement.

Swiss chard also is a great candidate as a raw food. Blend it in a smoothie with some cantaloupe or apple to sweeten and add a tablespoon of palm oil to help absorb the carotenes from the chard.

Tuna

Tuna is an excellent source of high-quality protein with a low calorie count. It also is a good source of selenium, which is an anti-cancer agent. Six ounces of fresh tuna will provide 100 percent of your daily protein requirement, 100 percent of your selenium requirement, and 23 percent of your omega-3 requirement. The protein is high quality and a complete protein.

Tuna raises omega-3 levels in blood, which is great for your heart and joints. In a study by W. S. Harris[88], a small group of healthy women, all pre-menopausal in age, consumed a daily average of 485 milligrams of omega-3 fatty acids by either eating salmon and/or albacore tuna (both rich in omega-3 fats) twice a week or by taking one to two capsules of fish oil daily.

After 16 weeks, levels of omega-3s in their red blood cells were measured. In those eating fish, omega-3 levels increased from an average of 4.0 to 6.2 of total fatty acids. In those taking capsules, omega-3 levels rose virtually an identical amount, from 4.3 to 6.2 percent of total fatty acids. EPA in red blood cells increased significantly more rapidly in the fish group than in the capsule group during the first four weeks, but rates did not differ significantly between groups thereafter. It may be more beneficial to eat tuna rather than take capsules.

The media is replete with scare-tactic stories about mercury in seafood — they love the hype. The truth is: If you have adequate vitamin C intake, then your body can prevent accumulation of mercury, cadmium and lead, as the vitamin C chelates the heavy metals. Millions of people per year are dying of heart disease and cancer, yet, have you lately heard of anyone dying from mercury poisoning? The omega-3 and selenium in tuna are potent preventers of cancer and heart disease. Mercury toxicity is a symptom of vitamin C deficiency, NOT eating too much tuna. For the ability of vitamin C to prevent mercury toxicity, see Irwin Stone[89].

Turmeric — Super Food

Turmeric has been given super food status because of its powerful anti-inflammatory properties. It has one of the highest ORAC values of all foods known, only cloves, the highest at 314,000 units per 100 grams and cinnamon (266,000 units per 100 grams) are higher than turmeric at 159,000 units per 100 grams. Among many of its benefits, turmeric:

Treats bowel diseases.
Treats cystic fibrosis.
Prevents breast cancer.
Cures polyps in bowel.
Treats prostate cancer.
Prevents arterial plaque.

Although it is a spice and used in small quantities, one-half teaspoon will add 1,600 ORAC units to any meal. Experts recommend at least 5,000 ORAC units per day in the diet.

Curcumin, the active ingredient in turmeric, has been shown to treat inflammatory bowel disease, Crohns disease, breast cancer, polyps in human colons, prevented the free-radical damage that causes plaque in the arteries, and retarded the growth of prostate cancer cells. And when used in combination with *isothiocyanate*, (from cruciferous vegetables) it stopped the growth of prostate cancer cells altogether (A. T. Kong)[90]. It also was found effective in protecting the brain against Alzheimer's disease.

Instead of using curry, try turmeric, depending on the recipe. Curry powder may not have much turmeric in it. We suggest you keep turmeric powder in the kitchen and add it to meat, rice, beans, etc., at the rate of one-half teaspoon per meal. Add turmeric after the food is cooked.

Watercress — Super Food

For the remarkable anti-cancer benefits of watercress, see Chapter 4: Why Raw is Better. As it usually is eaten raw, the anti-cancer substances are released as opposed to cooking, which would interfere with this process. However, cooking recipes do exist and, if cooked, it should be done extremely lightly.

Watercress is elevated to super food status because it does not suppress thyroid action like the other cruciferous foods and because it usually is eaten raw. As a matter of fact, its iodine content boosts thyroid output. So if you have low thyroid output and cannot eat cruciferous vegetables, you can get this cancer benefit from eating watercress. The iodine in watercress is the right quantity mixed with other healthful substances.

If you have thyroid problems, such as palpitations or enlargement of the gland itself, you should eat watercress on a regular basis. You will find it a great remedy if you lack vitality and are always listless and tired — both symptoms usually caused by the poor function of the endocrine glands. In addition, its mineral, iron and iodine content stimulate glandular activity. Iodine also has been found to be a factor in decreasing breast cancer.

Watercress contains 103 percent of the daily vitamin C requirement, 53 percent of the vitamin A requirement and 15 percent of the daily vitamin E content — all in only 100 grams! See Chapter 10 for a delicious recipe: Watercress and Berry Salad.

Watermelon

Watermelon has almost twice as much lycopene as tomatoes, which are commonly touted as the best source of lycopene. Watermelon has 4,532 micrograms per 100 grams, compared to tomatoes with 2,570 micrograms per 100 grams. Lycopene in tomatoes can be concentrated by drying or turning into sauces. But tomatoes are in the nightshade family, which means there are substances in it that make joints stiff and painful for individuals susceptible to arthritis. This makes watermelon a good source of lycopene for such persons and, in general, we can eat a lot more watermelon than tomatoes in one sitting.

In numerous studies, lycopene has been shown to inhibit the formation of prostate cancer (P.H. Gann[91]). And while we point out that the major role of copper-containing superoxide dismutase (SOD) is destroying free radicals that cause cancer, lycopene helps destroy them too.

Wheat Bran (Unrefined)

Wheat bran is the material that is removed from the outer layer of the wheat when it is refined or turned into white flour. The bran contains much of the nutrients in the whole kernel. One cup or two ounces of bran contains 25 grams of fiber, which is our complete daily requirement. It also contains 6.7 milligrams of manganese, which is 333 percent of our requirement!

We point out repeatedly the effects of copper and manganese in the body and their role in the health of the cell, but we can't say it enough. Cancer cells low in copper and manganese (SOD), benefit when the levels of copper and manganese are corrected in the cell, which can return the cell to normal.

Brans are loaded with omega-6 fatty acids, approximately 8,000 milligrams per 100 grams. Having no omega-3 fatty acids (or almost none), brans need to be balanced with high omega-3 foods. Your 100-gram serving of bran also contains 18 percent of your daily protein requirement, 30 percent of copper, 34 percent of iron, and it only contains about 125 calories.

Yogurt

Yogurt contains friendly bacteria of the *lactobacillus* family, which combats disease-causing bacteria not just in the bowel, but in the whole body.

Yogurt has been found to aid in the treatment of yeast infections, reduce the incidence of ulcers, and it even reduces the inflammation of arthritis. The best type of yogurt contains live organisms, although even killed organisms have been found to have immune-stimulatory effects.

Recipes for Healthy, Disease-Free Living

CHAPTER 10

Using the knowledge and ideas found in this book, enjoy the delicious tastes of your favorite foods, and find pleasure in some new favorites — simultaneously enhancing your overall health and wellness.

These delicious recipes will help you incorporate the health benefits of raw ingredients and gluten-free foods and add an abundance of fruits and vegetables to your meals. And no matter your family size, these recipe amounts easily can be increased or decreased to fit your needs.

Be versatile, experiment with different foods and flavors and ignite your taste buds, all with the help and guidance of "Eat Right for Life!"

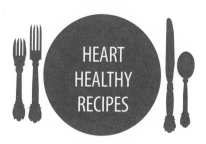

HEART
HEALTHY
RECIPES

Summer Slaw for Two

INGREDIENTS
Half of one fresh cabbage, grated
2 carrots, grated
4 tablespoons flax seed, olive or safflower oil
1 lemon, juiced
Sea salt to taste
2 ounces red raisins or 4 ounces fresh red grapes
2 teaspoons fresh parsley, chopped
2 teaspoons fresh cilantro, chopped
2 teaspoons fresh basil, chopped (optional)

DIRECTIONS
Combine all ingredients and mix well. Refrigerate.

BENEFITS
Supplies potent anti-cancer enzymes, substances and carotenes.
Contains omega-3 and/or omega-9, which helps prevent heart disease , cancer and arthritis.
Provides vitamin C, which boosts the immune system and strengthens bones.
Contains red resveratrol, which helps prevent heart disease and helps to control and reverse the signs of aging.
Rich in essential nutrients and anti-oxidants.
Helps neutralize carcinogens.
Removes heavy metals, such as mercury, from the body.

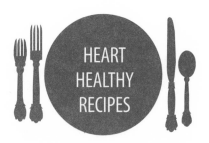

HEART
HEALTHY
RECIPES

Terrific Tuna Salad for Two

INGREDIENTS
6-ounce can tuna
2 tablespoons flax seed oil
1 egg, boiled and chopped
1/4 onion, finely chopped
1 squeeze fresh lemon juice
Sea salt to taste

DIRECTIONS
Combine all ingredients and mix well. Refrigerate.

BENEFITS
Provides complete protein, zinc and copper, which promote cardiovascular health and boosts the immune system.
Contains omega-3 and/or omega 9, which helps prevent cancer, heart disease and arthritis.
Provides vitamin C, which boosts the immune system and strengthens bones.
Great source of daily vitamins and protein.
Stimulates growth of healthy bacteria in the colon and has been found to reduce rates of stomach cancer.

According to an article written by Eric Margolis and published in the Toronto Sun, "Americans, who comprise only 5 percent of the world's population, account for a whopping 33 percent of total global sugar consumption - over 10 million tons annually".

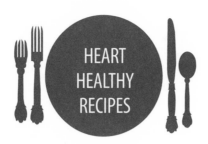

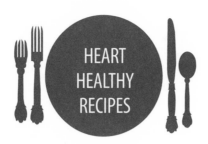

Faux Mashed Potatoes (Cauliflower Puree)

INGREDIENTS
1 medium raw head of cauliflower
Salt and pepper to taste
Milk, butter, or cream (enough to make it creamy, same as making mashed potatoes)
*Optional: 2 fresh cloves or 2 teaspoons minced garlic

DIRECTIONS
Break the cauliflower into florets. Steam the cauliflower until it is tender (it is ready when a fork can easily pierce the floret). Using a potato masher or blender, start to add in milk, butter or cream until your desired consistency is reached. Optional: Mash or blend in fresh or minced garlic. Serve and enjoy!

BENEFITS
High in glucosinolates (anti-cancer compounds, famous in cruciferous vegetables.
Vegetarian friendly.
Gluten free
Low carbohydrate.
Free of nightshade family compounds that aggravate arthritis.

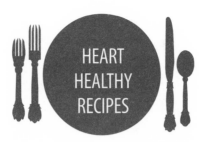

HEART
HEALTHY
RECIPES

Biltong (South African Jerky)

INGREDIENTS
Beef
Coriander powder
*Optional: Black pepper to taste
Vinegar (enough to cover beef while soaking)
Sea salt (to taste)

DIRECTIONS
Remove beef sinews with sharp kitchen scissors then cut raw beef into thin strips. The longer the strip, the easier it is to handle; the thinner the strip the quicker it dries. Soak the beef in vinegar for at least 10 minutes. On a clean counter, liberally apply sea salt to both sides of the meat. Dust the meat with coriander powder (if desired, black pepper can also be used). Make hooks from metal paper clips by bending them open. Use the hooks to hang the meat from a rod or dowel (lay old towels under the hanging meat to catch any drips). Aim a fan at the meat to move the air and aid in the drying process. The jerky will be done after approximately two days, although if you prefer a different texture you can let it dry longer.
The warmer the air, the quicker the jerky will dry, but even in cool air it eventually will dry. For those concerned about the meat spoiling, vinegar preserves the meat. And once the vinegar is evaporated, the salt and lack of moisture preserves the meat.

Important Tips

DO NOT dry meat in an outside unscreened area. Yellow jackets (hornets) and flies are especially drawn to meat, especially raw meat. If you do not have an appropriate place to hang your raw jerky, you can purchase a food dehydrator. However, be careful to keep the temperature as low as possible as they generate hot air and may slightly "cook" the food.
**You can also use food dehydrators to dehydrate fruits and vegetables, make natural fruit leathers, and other healthy take-a-long snacks that pack a nutritional punch!

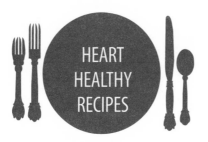

HEART
HEALTHY
RECIPES

BENEFITS

Avoids the cooking process, which kills many of the meats nutritional properties.

Vinegar digests the protein and also temporally preserves the meat (the darker the red vinegar, the higher the anti-oxidant value.

Salt permanently preserves the meat, making and keeping it safe to eat and store naturally.

Salt also provides electrolytes and makes hydrochloric acid in the stomach, which digests protein.

Coriander provides anti-oxidants and flavor.

Pepper stimulates and improves digestion.

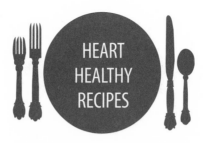

HEART
HEALTHY
RECIPES

Kombu Stock

INGREDIENTS
6 cups of water
6-inch piece dried kombu

DIRECTIONS
Cut the piece of kombu lengthwise and then cut the long pieces into 1-inch pieces.
Soak kombu in a pot of water for 15 to 20 minutes. Then, bring water to a simmer over medium heat and simmer for 5 minutes.
Remove the kombu and store in the refrigerator. When reusing kombu to make stock, bring water to a boil, add the kombu and reduce heat to simmer for 15 to 20 minutes. Cutting the kombu pieces in half will help release the amino acids that make up the flavor. Remove kombu and store in refrigerator.

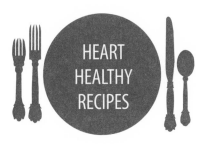

Hearty Kombu Miso Soup

INGREDIENTS
4 cups kombu stock
1 cup vegetable broth
3 carrots cut thinly
1 cup cooked brown rice noodles
1/4 cup frozen peas
2 tablespoons non-gmo miso
1/4 cup scallions, cut into ¼-inch pieces
1 tablespoon soy sauce or sea salt to taste
3 tablespoons fresh cilantro
Optional: 1 garlic clove
Optional: 1-inch julienned precooked kombu

DIRECTIONS
Heat kombu stock and vegetable broth in quart pot and add the carrots. Simmer for 10 minutes or until carrots can be pierced with a fork. Turn off heat. Ladle some of the stock into a small bowl and stir in miso until smooth. Add back into the soup pot and stir. Stir in all the other ingredients and you are ready to serve.

BENEFITS
A powerful source of iodine, anti-cancer and thyroid support.
The iodine is in a form readily usable by the thyroid gland.

Tip
For a thicker luscious soup, cook the rice noodles in the kombu and vegetable stock with the carrots. Then turn stove off and proceed to add remaining ingredients.

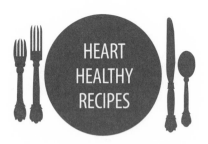

Lemon Grass Coconut Soup

INGREDIENTS
3 cups of water
6 thin slices fresh ginger
1 stem lemon grass, slice thin (about 3 inches)
1 carrot, thinly slice on the diagonal
1 garlic clove, mince
1 dash cayenne pepper
1 teaspoon sea salt
1 yellow zucchini, slice thin
1 tablespoon crushed coriander seeds
2 cups sliced mushrooms, white, crimini or baby bella
1/2 cup peas, fresh or frozen
14-ounce can coconut milk (light or regular)
1 lemon or lime (squeezed)
3 tablespoons chopped cilantro

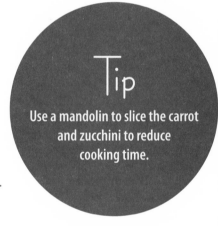

Tip
Use a mandolin to slice the carrot and zucchini to reduce cooking time.

DIRECTIONS
Start with 3 cups of water in a quart-size pot over medium heat. Toss in sliced ginger and lemon grass. When water comes to a low boil, add carrot, garlic, cayenne pepper and sea salt. Add the zucchini and crushed coriander seeds as well as the sliced mushrooms. Simmer for a few minutes until mushrooms are slightly tender and then add peas and coconut milk. Stir and turn off heat. Add lemon juice and fresh cilantro. Add a second dash of cayenne pepper if you desire a hotter soup. Serve and enjoy.

BENEFITS
Mushrooms have powerful immuno-stimulatory and liver protective effects.
Ginger and lemon grass have good amounts of anti-oxidants
Lemongrass, as pointed out in the cancer section, in Chapter 1, is known for killing cancer cells.

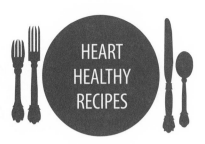

Lebanese Salad (Fattoush)

SALAD INGREDIENTS
1 cup thin-sliced toasted bread broken into small pieces
3 medium-size cucumbers, dice, peel and remove seeds if necessary
3 large Roma tomatoes or one large regular tomato
4 scallions
1/2 cup chopped Italian parsley
1/2 cup chopped mint leaves

DRESSING INGREDIENTS
1/4 cup fresh lime or lemon juice
2 garlic cloves, mince
1 teaspoon ground cumin
2 teaspoons ground sumac
1/2 teaspoon sea salt
1/2 teaspoon red pepper flakes or dash of cayenne pepper
3 tablespoons extra-virgin olive oil
Optional: Fresh ground black pepper to taste

DIRECTIONS
Toss vegetables in salad bowl. Combine salad dressing in separate container. Just before serving, mix in salad dressing and toasted bread. Serve immediately so bread does not become soggy.

BENEFITS
Parsley provides vitamin C, the anti-infection vitamin, plus anti-tumor compounds.
Cucumber is an excellent source of silica, for a stronger body and healthier skin.
Mint soothes the stomach.

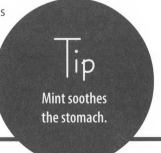

Tip
Mint soothes
the stomach.

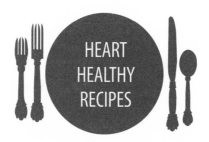

HEART
HEALTHY
RECIPES

Simple Green Olive Tapenade

INGREDIENTS
2 cups pitted green olives or 16-ounce can pitted green olives in salt water (drain and rinse)
1 clove garlic, cut in small pieces or mince
1/2 teaspoon lime or lemon zest
2 teaspoons finely chopped parsley
2 tablespoons extra-virgin olive oil
1/2 cup walnut halves

DIRECTIONS
Toast walnut halves in a cast iron skillet; remove from heat and let cool. Pour toasted walnuts in food processor and blend on medium for two seconds (just into small chunks, not enough to turn into a flour). Remove from processor and set aside. Put all ingredients, except olive oil and walnuts, in food processor and pulse until thoroughly pureed. Add olive oil and pulse until incorporated. Add walnuts and process on low until thoroughly mixed. Serve and enjoy.

BENEFITS
Olives are a source of vitamin E, iron and anti-oxidants.
Walnuts are a source of the critical nutrient copper, which makes SOD that prevents cancer and heart disease.

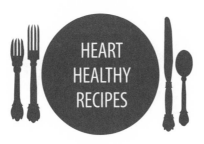

HEART
HEALTHY
RECIPES

Herring (Pickled Fish)

INGREDIENTS
3 quarts raw wild herring, skinned, filleted and cut into small pieces
1 quart water
1 cup canning salt
1 quart vinegar
2 bay leaves
2 teaspoons pickling spices
1 cup Rhine wine
2 cups (or more) sliced onions
Optional: Sour cream to taste

DIRECTIONS
Place herring in a glass jar or bowl. Heat 1 quart water and 1 cup canning salt, then cool. When cool, pour the water/salt mixture over the fish and cover with a glass plate or jar cover. Leave sit for 24 hours in the refrigerator. Remove from fridge, rinse well and set aside. In a stainless steel pot, boil 1 quart vinegar, 2 teaspoons pickling spices and 2 bay leaves. When cool, pour 1 cup Rhine wine over the fish and add lots of sliced onions. If desired, add some sour cream.
Put fish in jars, cover and let stand in refrigerator for 3 to 4 days. Eat and enjoy!

BENEFITS
Benefits of raw food — a powerful source of omega-3 fatty acids, vitamin D and selenium, all cancer and heart disease-preventing nutrients.
Great source of vitamin B12, the anti-anemic vitamin.

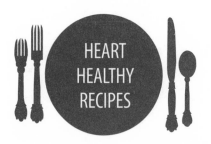

Supa'- Dupa' HGH Protein Drink (FOR AFTER EXERCISE)

INGREDIENTS
1 glass raw milk
3 raw organic high omega-3 eggs
1 tablespoon blackstrap molasses

DIRECTIONS
Put in blender and mix. Molasses can be varied to taste, but more provides more minerals.
Pour into glass — bottoms up!

BENEFITS
Supplies your body with arginine and glutamine, vitamin A, copper, selenium and manganese.
Raw food supplies protein required to make human growth hormone (HGH).
Completely natural compared to those questionable protein powders.

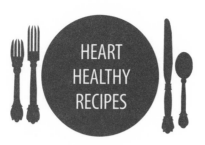

HEART
HEALTHY
RECIPES

Homemade Yellow Mustard

INGREDIENTS
1/2 cup yellow mustard seeds
3/4 cup raw apple cider vinegar
1/3 cup water
2 teaspoons turmeric
1 clove garlic, peel and crush

DIRECTIONS
Soak the mustard seeds in the vinegar and water, making sure the seeds are covered by the liquid. Leave soak for 2 days. After 2 days of soaking has passed, add the turmeric and garlic to the seeds mixture. Blend mixture until it reaches desired consistency, adding water if needed. Store in the refrigerator.

BENEFITS
Potent source of the isothiocyanates found in cruciferous vegetables.
Turmeric is a powerful source of anti-oxidants.
All of these ingredients conspire to provide immunity against cancer and heart disease.

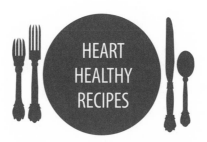

Rooibos Tea

INGREDIENTS
1 large cup water
2 spoonfuls or tea bags Rooibos tea leaves
2 pieces star aniseed
1 cinnamon stick
3 to 4 whole cloves
Small orange slice

DIRECTIONS
Steep the tea leaves, star aniseed, cinnamon stick and cloves until you have reached your desired tea darkness. Add the orange slice and enjoy. For those on the go, you can get vanilla rooibos at Starbucks!

BENEFITS
Powerful anti-oxidants.

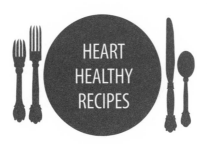

HEART
HEALTHY
RECIPES

Yucca Cuban Mojo

INGREDIENTS:
1/2 pound yucca root, halve and cut into chunks
1 teaspoon salt
Juice of 1 lime
6 garlic cloves, mash
1 teaspoon salt
1/3 cup fresh lemon juice
1/2 cup olive oil
1 onion, chop fine

DIRECTIONS
Place yucca in saucepan; add salt and lime juice and bring to a boil. Reduce heat, cover and simmer until tender, about 30 minutes. Drain and keep warm. Mash garlic cloves into salt with mortar and pestle (or use food processor). In a separate pan, add olive oil, mashed garlic, lemon juice, and onions. Heat until bubbling, then pour over yucca. Toss yucca and sauce "lightly" cooking to sauté over medium heat until barely brown but not crisp.

BENEFITS
According to folk medicine, yucca extracts have anti-arthritic and anti-inflammatory effects.
Protozoa are small micro-organisms that can be seen in water under a microscope. They can cause infections and serious diseases. Yucca has a substance in it that can kill protozoa.
It has been postulated that yucca may have anti-arthritic properties by suppressing intestinal protozoa, which may have a role in joint inflammation.
It is a rich source of anti-oxidants including resveratrol and a number of yucca compounds. These have anti-inflammatory activity. Yucca phenolics are also anti-oxidants and free-radical scavengers, which may aid in suppressing reactive oxygen species that stimulate inflammatory responses such as arthritis and atherosclerosis.

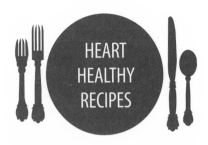

HEART
HEALTHY
RECIPES

Basil Cilantro Pesto

INGREDIENTS
1 bunch fresh basil
1 bunch fresh cilantro
1 cup walnuts
2/3 cup water
Juice of 1 lime
1/2 teaspoon salt

DIRECTIONS
In a food processor, put in basil, cilantro and water. Process until blended. Add lime juice, salt and walnuts. Blend until smooth. Store in an airtight container and refrigerate. Use on meats, rice, pasta or veggie burgers.

BENEFITS
Basil and cilantro are powerful sources of anti-oxidants.
Walnuts are a powerful source of minerals especially copper and manganese that make the enzyme superoxide dismutase (SOD).

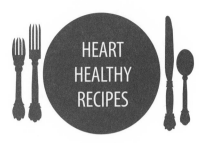

HEART
HEALTHY
RECIPES

Almond Milk

Ingredients
1/2 cup raw almonds
4 cups water
Optional: 2 tablespoons organic raisins

DIRECTIONS
Put all ingredients in a blender. Blend on high speed until smooth, adding more water for desired level of consistency. You can strain the milk. Place a fine mesh sieve over a bowl. Slowly stir the milk with a spatula, which helps it pass more quickly. Be sure to keep the milk refrigerated.

BENEFITS
A powerful source of minerals, especially copper and manganese that make SOD, an enzyme that prevents cells from becoming cancerous, strengthens arteries and prevents plaque.

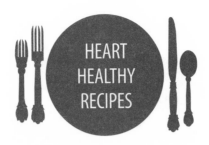

Almond Milk With Blackstrap Molasses

INGREDIENTS
1/2 cup raw almonds
4 cups water
Optional: 2 tablespoons organic raisins
2 tablespoons unsulfered blackstrap molasses

DIRECTIONS
Blend all ingredients on high speed until smooth. You can add more water and blend again to your preferred consistency.

BENEFITS
Almonds and blackstrap molasses are a powerful source of minerals, especially copper and manganese that make SOD, an enzyme that prevents cells from becoming cancerous, strengthens arteries and prevents plaque.

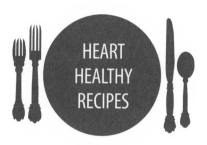

HEART HEALTHY RECIPES

Lima Bean Dip or Mock Avocado Dip

INGREDIENTS
3 cups cooked lima beans, fresh or frozen
1/4 cup lemon or lime juice
1 minced garlic clove (or more to taste)
2 tablespoons fresh cilantro
1 tablespoon safflower oil
2 tablespoons fresh chopped parsley
1/2 teaspoon ground cumin
1/2 teaspoon cayenne pepper
1/4 teaspoon dried coriander

DIRECTIONS
Puree ingredients in a food processor until smooth. Chill to desired coolness.

BENEFITS
Spices and greens are powerful sources of anti-oxidants.
Safflower oil supplies omega-9 fatty acids, similar to omega-3 fatty acids.

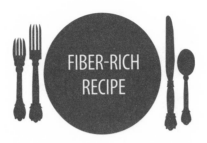

FIBER-RICH
RECIPE

Simple Chicken Pasta Salad

INGREDIENTS
4 ounces cooked whole-wheat pasta, twists or bows
6 ounces baked boneless chicken breast, cube or shred
1 cup fresh chopped broccoli
1/2 cup fresh or frozen peas
Diced tomatoes (to taste)
1 teaspoon Italian blend herbs
1/4 teaspoon white pepper
1 tablespoon fresh grated Parmesan cheese

DIRECTIONS
Combine all ingredients in salad bowl, cover and chill for 20 minutes.

BENEFITS
Whole-wheat pasta supplies fiber, vitamins and minerals.
Chicken supplies protein.
Broccoli offers anti-cancer substances.

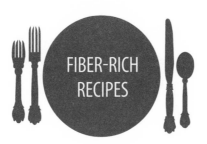

FIBER-RICH
RECIPES

Easy Brown Rice and Beans

INGREDIENTS
4 tablespoons brown rice
3/4 cup water
7-ounce can stewed tomatoes
1/3 cup chopped celery (1 stalk)
1/3 cup chopped onions (1/2 medium onion)
1/2 cup chopped green peppers (1/2 medium pepper)
7 ounces cooked red kidney beans
1/2 clove fresh garlic, mince
Dash of pepper
Optional: 2 drops hot sauce

DIRECTIONS
Cook rice according to package directions. In skillet, cook chopped celery, onion, and green peppers over low heat for 10 minutes. Add red beans, stewed tomatoes and seasoning. Bring to a boil, then simmer uncovered about 10 minutes. Mix in cooked rice, then serve and enjoy.

BENEFITS
Brown rice is a whole source of fiber, minerals and vitamins.
Beans supply fiber and protein.
Tomatoes supply anti-cancer lycophene.

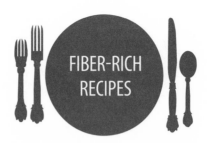

FIBER-RICH
RECIPES

Black Bean Hummus

Ingredients
1 clove garlic
15-ounce can black beans, drain and reserve liquid
2 tablespoons lemon juice
1-1/2 tablespoons tahini
3/4 teaspoon ground cumin
1/2 teaspoon salt
1/4 teaspoon cayenne pepper
1/4 teaspoon paprika
10 Greek olives

DIRECTIONS
Mince garlic in the bowl of a food processor. Add black beans, 2 tablespoons reserved bean liquid, lemon juice, tahini, cumin, salt and cayenne pepper. Process until smooth, scraping down the sides as needed. Add additional seasoning and liquid to taste. Garnish with paprika and Greek olives.

BENEFITS
Beans supply protein and fiber.
Tahini is a powerful source of copper and manganese.
Olives supply anti-oxidants.
All this provides immunity to cancer and heart disease.

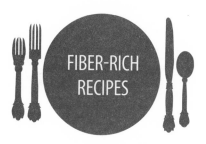

FIBER-RICH
RECIPES

Butternut Squash Soup

INGREDIENTS
2 teaspoons olive oil
2 medium onions, chop
3 to 4 garlic cloves, mince
1 large butternut squash, peel and cube
3 to 4 potatoes, peel and cube
3/4 cup unsweetened apple juice (make sure it's 100 percent juice)
3-1/4 cups chicken or vegetable broth
1/2 cup soy or rice milk
1 teaspoon ginger
3 tablespoons fresh chopped parsley, divided

DIRECTIONS
In a large soup pot, sauté onions and garlic in olive oil for 3 to 5 minutes. Add squash, potatoes, juice and broth and bring to a boil. Reduce heat and simmer 40 to 45 minutes. Mash a few pieces of squash and potatoes against side of pot to ensure they are soft. Ladle half of the mixture into a food processor or blender and purée. Add puréed mixture back into pot. Add milk, ginger and 2 teaspoons of parsley. Simmer for 3 to 5 minutes. Top with remaining teaspoon of parsley and serve warm.

BENEFITS
Butternut squash is a whopping source of vitamin A; supplies some manganese.
Ginger and parsley are high sources of anti-oxidants.
Onion and garlic are good for cardiovascular health.

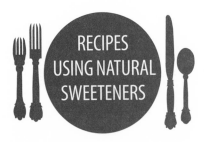

RECIPES USING NATURAL SWEETENERS

Super Healthy Natural Breakfast Cereal (DELICIOUS TOO)

INGREDIENTS
1 cup raw buckwheat groats
1/3 cup chia seeds
1/2 cup cashew nut pieces
1 tablespoon blackstrap molasses, add more or less to taste
1 cup raw milk or unsweetened rice, almond, or soy milk

DIRECTIONS
Mix all ingredients and enjoy!

BENEFITS
Starts your day out well with anti-cancer and heart disease-fighting nutrients.
Protein from the buckwheat and the chia is high quality; meal will supply approximately 50 percent of your daily protein requirement.
Relatively low-calorie load at 600 to 700 calories.

Tip
This cereal is quite crunchy and must be well-chewed — good for stimulating your gums and relieving stress.

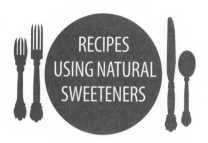

Banana Molasses Cookies

INGREDIENTS
1/2 cup buckwheat flour
3/4 cup brown rice flour
1 teaspoon baking powder
1/2 teaspoon cinnamon
1/2 teaspoon ginger
1/4 teaspoon cloves
1/8 teaspoon salt
1/2 mashed banana
1/2 cup maple syrup
6 tablespoons safflower oil
2 tablespoons blackstrap molasses

DIRECTIONS
Preheat oven to 325 F. In a mixing bowl, stir together buckwheat and brown-rice flours, baking powder, cinnamon, ginger, cloves and salt. In a second bowl, mix maple syrup, vegetable oil, molasses, and mashed banana. Add flour mixture to maple syrup mixture and stir until mixed. Using a tablespoon, scoop up dough and form nice mounds. Place the mounds about 2-½ inches apart on a greased cookie sheet. Bake for 13 to 16 minutes. Let cool for 2 minutes on sheet, then transfer to a wire rack to cool. Makes about 18 cookies

BENEFITS
Buckwheat is a huge source of rutin and bioflavonoids, which are anti-oxidants that help circulation and prevent heart disease.

Whole rice supplies fiber mineral and B vitamins.
Cinnamon, ginger and cloves are powerful sources of the anti-oxidants that make cells resistant to cancer.
Maple syrup is a whole sweetener.
Blackstrap molasses is a concentrated source of the minerals that make cells strong and resistant to cancer and a natural sweetener.

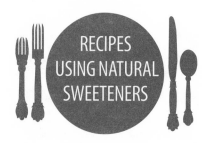

RECIPES
USING NATURAL
SWEETENERS

Golden Cream Cookies

CRUST INGREDIENTS
1 cup walnut or almond meal (ground nuts)
1/2 cup date sugar
1/3 cup water

FILLING INGREDIENTS
8 ounces cream cheese, softened
1/2 cup maple syrup
1/2 banana
1/2 teaspoon orange zest
1/2 teaspoon lime zest
Fresh berries and mint leaves for garnish

DIRECTIONS
Preheat oven to 350 F. Combine nut meal, water and date sugar in food processor.
Press dough into a parchment lined 8-inch glass pan. Bake for 5 minutes. For filling,
blend cheese, maple syrup, banana and zests together in processor until smooth. Pour
over crust. Bake for 25 to 30 minutes. Cool completely. Cut into squares before serving.
Decorate tops with berries and mint leaves.

BENEFITS
Walnut and almond meal are a rich source of copper and manganese that make anti-
oxidant anti-cancer enzymes in the body.
Date sugar and maple syrup are holistic replacements for white sugar.

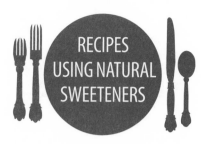

RECIPES USING NATURAL SWEETENERS

Citrus Cookies

INGREDIENTS
1/4 cup safflower oil
8 ounces cream cheese, room temperature
3/4 cup maple syrup
1/4 teaspoon salt
1 teaspoon lime or lemon zest
2 teaspoons orange zest
Juice of 1 lime
2 tablespoons water
2 cups whole rice flour
1 tablespoon baking powder
Walnut halves for tops of cookies

DIRECTIONS
Preheat oven to 325 F. Cream together the oil, cream cheese, maple syrup, water, lime juice, zest and salt. Beat well. Stir in the flour mixture. Shape cookie dough into small round balls and flatten slightly with palm of hand. Place onto lightly oiled baking sheet then press a walnut half into the top of each. Bake for 20 to 25 minutes or until tops of cookies have been risen in center for 5 minutes. Remove cookies to a rack to cool. Makes over 2 dozen cookies.

BENEFITS
Safflower oil is rich in the anti-cancer omega-9 fatty acids.
Maple syrup is a holistic replacement for the refined white sugar.
Rice flour is a gluten-free replacement for flour.

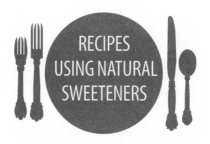

RECIPES
USING NATURAL
SWEETENERS

Almond Rose Cookies

INGREDIENTS
1/2 cup safflower oil
1/2 cup maple syrup
1 egg, or equivalent egg substitute
2 teaspoons Rose water (Any Mediterranean or Persian store will have Rose water)
1 cup plus 2 tablespoons brown rice flour
1 cup ground almonds (almond meal)
1 teaspoon baking powder
1/4 teaspoon sea salt

DIRECTIONS
Preheat oven to 400 F. In medium bowl, whisk together the oil and syrup. Beat in egg or substitute. Stir in Rose water. In another bowl, mix together the flour, almond meal, baking powder and sea salt. Blend with a pastry blender. Add wet ingredients to the dry and stir until flour is moistened. Drop by teaspoonfuls 2 inches apart on lightly greased cookie sheets. Bake 10 to 15 minutes, checking for cookies to be golden on the edges. Remove and let cool on rack or wooden cutting board. Makes about 2 dozen.

BENEFITS
Safflower oil is high in the anti-cancer omega-9 fatty acids.
Almond meal is rich in copper and manganese, which makes the anti-cancer and anti-heart disease superoxide dismutase (SOD) for cells in the body.
Brown rice supplies minerals and vitamins.
Rose fragrance uplifts the mind and spirit.

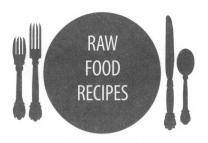

RAW
FOOD
RECIPES

Sweet Carrot Pate´

INGREDIENTS
3 large raw carrots, cut into 2-inch pieces
1/2 cup raw almonds
1/4 cup raisins
1/2 teaspoon cardamom
Juice of 1/2 lemon or lime
1/4 cup water

DIRECTIONS
Blend all ingredients together on high speed blender. Spoon into tiny bowls and serve.

BENEFITS
Carrots supply vitamin A, an anti-cancer vitamin.
Almonds supply copper and manganese; anti-cancer minerals make SOD.

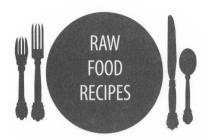

RAW
FOOD
RECIPES

Super Green Smoothie

INGREDIENTS
1 cup melon, cantaloupe or watermelon (or 1 cup grapes)
1 banana
1/2 to 1 cup water (your desired thickness)
2 handfuls of baby spinach
1 tablespoon acerola cherry powder
1 tablespoon blackstrap molasses
2 tablespoons chia seeds
1/2 teaspoon turmeric powder
2 tablespoons red palm oil

DIRECTIONS
Blend fruit and water on medium to high speed in blender. Add greens, blend. Set blender to low, and slowly add remaining ingredients. Blend a few seconds at high speed. Pour into 16-ounce glass and drink. Mix your greens and fruits for a variety of flavors and get a great start to the day.

BENEFITS
Loaded with anti-oxidants and minerals, especially copper.
Palm oil is a whopping source of vitamin A.
Your body will rejoice when fed this stuff!

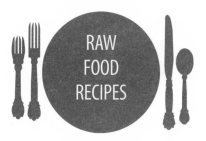

Cucumbers and Spicy Mint Sauce

INGREDIENTS
3 cucumbers, wash and slice
1 bunch mint, remove stems
Dash cayenne pepper or to taste
1 teaspoon salt
2 tablespoons olive oil
2 tablespoons balsamic vinegar
2 tablespoons grape molasses (check online or at Greek deli) or maple syrup

DIRECTIONS
Wash the fresh mint leaves (without stems). In a food processor, add mint leaves, salt, oil, vinegar and syrup and blend well until it looks consistent with tiny pieces. Spoon enough over cucumbers and serve immediately. Store remainder of mint sauce in refrigerator.

BENEFITS
Mint soothes the stomach, has anti-tumor agents and anti-asthma properties.

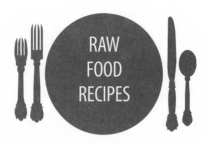

RAW
FOOD
RECIPES

Tricolor Cole Slaw

INGREDIENTS
1/2 head green cabbage
1/2 head red cabbage
2 shredded carrots
1/2 red onion, slice thin and chop
1/2 cup finely chopped Italian parsley
3 tablespoons finely chopped fresh basil
1 tablespoon maple syrup
1 teaspoon sea salt
1 dash cayenne pepper
1/2 cup lime or lemon juice
Optional: 1 teaspoon horseradish

DIRECTIONS
Shred or thinly slice the red and green cabbage in a large bowl. Add onion, parsley and basil to the bowl. Toss and mix evenly. Add remaining ingredients adjusting salt and pepper to taste. Serve and enjoy.

BENEFITS
Raw cabbage has powerful anti-cancer substances called isothiocyanates.

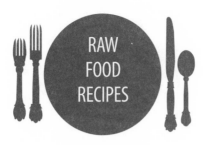

RAW
FOOD
RECIPES

Heavenly Raw-Fruit Pie

PIE CRUST INGREDIENTS
2-1/2 cups raw almonds
2 cups pitted dates

PIE FILLING INGREDIENTS
2 cups fresh cherries or strawberries
3 blood or navel oranges
2 to 3 bananas
1-1/2 cups blackberries or blueberries

CRUST DIRECTIONS
In a food processor, place almonds and process for 2 to 3 minutes or until the almonds are a medium fine meal. Add pitted dates, a few at a time, and process until all are blended and mixture comes together. In an 8-inch pie pan lined with parchment paper (parchment keeps the crust from adhering to the pan and makes it easy to serve), press the almond date mixture evenly on the bottom and up the sides of the pan. Refrigerate while preparing the fruit.

PIE FILLING DIRECTIONS
Trim strawberries and cut in half or, if using cherries, pit cherries and cut in half. Set aside. Take skins off oranges and slice thinly crosswise (through all sections) removing seeds. Set aside. Peel bananas and slice about 3/8-inch thick. Immediately layer over the pie crust (one layer). Take the sliced oranges and place over bananas. Try to cover all the banana slices. The juice of the orange will help keep the bananas from turning brown. Next layer the strawberries or cherries, cut-side down, over the orange layer. Line the outer edge of the pie with blackberries or blueberries and you're done. Chilling in the refrigerator for a few hours will give the citrus flavors time to meld into the other fruits and allow the pie crust time to harden a bit. Using a sharp knife, cut into pieces and then serve.

BENEFITS
A powerful combination of minerals (almonds) including the critical nutrient copper. Anti-oxidant-rich fruits.

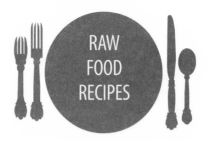

RAW
FOOD
RECIPES

Delicious Sweet-and-Sour Watercress Berry Salad

INGREDIENTS
3 cups fresh watercress, lightly washed and chopped
1 cup red grapes, the sweeter the better
1/2 of fresh lemon (or more, depending on your tastes)
1 half cup vegetable, olive or hemp seed oil
1/2 teaspoon turmeric
Salt to taste
Pepper to taste

DIRECTIONS
Combine watercress and grapes in a bowl. Sprinkle lemon juice over the watercress and grapes; toss. Add the oil and mix (we prefer hempseed oil, but olive oil also is good). Sprinkle mixture with salt, turmeric and pepper.
If the lemon juice is too sour for you, it can be diluted with an equal amount of water.

BENEFITS
Watercress contains strong anti-cancer sulforaphanes and iodine support for the thyroid.
Grapes supply anti-oxidants such as resveratrol.
Hempseed has a good ratio (2 to 1) of omega-6 to omega-3 and 9 fatty acids; inhibits breast cancer.
Olive oil contains omega-9 fatty acids.

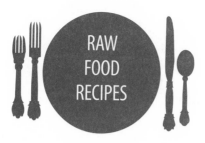

RAW FOOD RECIPES

Raw Pumpkin Seed Pesto

INGREDIENTS
1 cup raw pumpkin seeds
1/2 cup fresh basil
1/2 cup fresh cilantro
4 tablespoons fresh lime juice
1 garlic clove, minced
2 tablespoons olive oil
1/4 to 1/2 cup water (enough to process)
Salt to taste (1/4 to 1/2 teaspoon)
Dash of cayenne, if desired

DIRECTIONS
Mix together all the ingredients in a blender. Pulse until well blended. Store in airtight container. When ready to use, mix with your favorite vegetable pasta made from raw zucchini or other squash.

BENEFITS
The recipe amount supplies the daily requirement for copper and manganese.
Basil and cilantro supply anti-oxidants.
Olive oil supplies omega-9 fatty acids, similar to omega-3 fatty acids.
All ingredients are anti-cancer anti-heart disease.

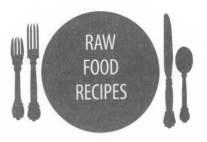

Cool Gazpacho
(RAW TOMATO SOUP)

INGREDIENTS
2 large heirloom tomatoes
1/2 large red bell pepper
1 large seedless cucumber
10 to 12 sprigs fresh cilantro
1/4 cup balsamic vinegar
Juice of 1 lime
Pinch of coriander
Dash of cayenne
1/4 teaspoon salt
1 clove garlic

DIRECTIONS
Cut tomatoes into chunks. Remove seeds from bell pepper and slice into 1-inch pieces. Cut cucumber into chunks with stem removed. Toss into food processor and blend until fairly smooth. Add in all remaining ingredients and blend. You're done! Serve with raw fresh corn on the cob. Makes 4 cups.

BENEFITS
A whopping dose of anti-cancer carotenes and anti-oxidants.
Cucumber provides silicon for healthier skin and stronger bones.

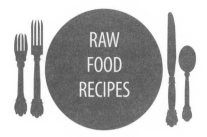

Sauerkraut (RAW)

INGREDIENTS

5 pounds cabbage, red or green (about two heads, preferably organic)
3-1/2 tablespoons coarse sea salt, unrefined (do not use iodized table salt)
1 gallon jar with glass lid
1 gallon plastic bucket
1 wooden dowel for crushing cabbage (ours is 2 feet long and 2 inches thick)
Some big stones, washed thoroughly (Make sure they will fit into the jar; used as weights. Or use another jar filled with water and sealed with a lid that fits nicely inside the gallon jar.)

DIRECTIONS

First, make sure that all dishes used for this project are very clean. Remove outer cabbage leaves and save three or four of the good looking leaves. Cut cabbage into quarter sections and remove the core. Shred cabbage into the width you desire and toss into clean bucket. Add salt and pound with mallet until water of cabbage releases. This takes about 15 to 20 minutes.
Place cabbage into jar and press down to the bottom with your fist, this helps remove air and make the liquid rise over the cabbage. Cabbage needs to be below the water so it does not come into contact with the air. If you need to add a little distilled or filtered water, do it now and sprinkle a little salt on top. Once you have all the cabbage pressed firmly down in the jar, place reserved cabbage leaves on top. Weight the cabbage down with your stones or heavy jar, making sure to keep cabbage below water line. Put lid on top and place in an undisturbed area. With glass jar you can check that the juices are always above the kraut. If you see a little foam in a few days, you can spoon this off the top. In about 1 week you can taste the sauerkraut and see if it is to your liking. Let it go longer if you want it to ripen more. When it is ready, you can remove large cabbage leaves and put shredded fermented cabbage and juice into clean airtight jars and refrigerate.

BENEFITS

A powerful anti-cancer food, supplying both isothiocyanates and additional anti-cancer substances from fermentation.
Red cabbage triples the amount of anti-oxidants and carotenes in this super food.

Tip

For a different and very delicious taste, add 2 quarter-size ginger slices and chopped and crushed green onion and garlic cloves when making the kraut.

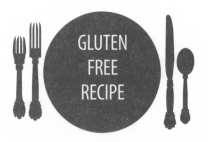

GLUTEN FREE RECIPE

Hoisin Sauce

INGREDIENTS
4 tablespoons wheat-free soy sauce
2 tablespoons almond butter
1 tablespoon blackstrap molasses
1 teaspoon maple syrup
2 teaspoons lemon juice
1/8 teaspoon garlic powder
2 teaspoons sesame oil
Pinch of cayenne (adjust for amount of hotness)

DIRECTIONS
Mix and use for dipping or drizzling over vegetables or meats.

BENEFITS:
Almonds and molasses are rich sources of copper, which makes the anti-oxidant SOD. Sesame oil is a good source of anti-inflammatory, anti-cancer omega-9 fatty acids.

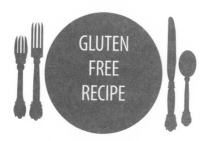

Go Crackers

INGREDIENTS
1 cup buckwheat flour
1 cup millet flour
1 cup almond meal
1 teaspoon sea salt
3 tablespoons unhulled sesame seeds
3 tablespoons dried garlic flakes
1 teaspoon fresh rosemary, chopped
4 tablespoons safflower oil
3/4 to 1 cup cold water
Parchment paper, size to fit inside baking sheet.
Salt and sesame seeds for sprinkling on top

Tip
Use other combinations of herbs like basil, cumin, cayenne or oregano. Experiment with other flours such as rice or oat flour or throw in some raw sunflower seeds. The crispness comes more from the almond meal so make sure you don't replace that ingredient when experimenting. If you want to use butter instead of safflower oil, go ahead. We use safflower oil to bake the crackers because it can take high heat. They are so easy to make.

DIRECTIONS
Preheat oven to 350 F. Mix dry ingredients in a large bowl so you can blend everything well. Add safflower oil and blend with pastry blender until mixed evenly. Add half of the water and mix. By this time you will probably want to start kneading with your hands. Add more water, little by little, and keep kneading until the dough comes together into a cohesive ball. Only use enough water to hold together, not sticky (this only takes a few minutes). Divide dough into even halves. On parchment paper press dough into oblong shape and start to roll with rolling pin from the center outward. You can also place a piece of parchment on top of dough before rolling if you prefer, but not necessary. Roll to 1/16-inch thick. Score the dough into squares or desired shape. Prick each square 2 or 3 times with a fork. Sprinkle sesame seeds and sea salt on top and press gently with rolling pin. Transfer parchment sheet of cracker dough to cookie sheet and bake 15 to 20 minutes or until golden brown. I find 20 minutes with whole flours works best. Turn baking sheet half way through baking time. Roll out second batch while first batch is baking. Let crackers cool before breaking apart. Store in airtight container. Makes about 3 cups of crackers.

BENEFITS
Two ounces of sesame seed will supply the daily requirement of the critical nutrient copper. High-oleic safflower oil is the best known source of anti-inflammatory anti-cancer omega-9.

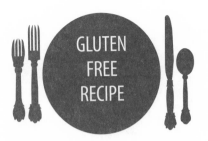

Black Bean Hummus

INGREDIENTS
2 cups cooked black beans
1/2 cup water
2 tablespoons fresh chopped cilantro
2 garlic cloves, mince
2 tablespoons fresh lemon or lime juice
2 tablespoon tahini (roasted sesame seed paste)
1 teaspoon ground cumin
1/4 teaspoon salt
Dash of crushed red pepper
2 teaspoons extra-virgin olive oil
Dash of ground red pepper
Salt, adjust to taste

DIRECTIONS
Place beans, water and garlic in a food processor; process until finely chopped. Add cilantro, lemon juice, tahini, cumin, salt and crushed red pepper; process until smooth. Spoon bean mixture into a medium bowl and drizzle with extra-virgin olive oil. Sprinkle with ground red pepper. Serve with corn chips or other gluten-free chips.

BENEFITS
The beans supply protein and fiber.
Tahini is a powerful source of copper and manganese.
Olives supply anti-oxidants.
Together they provide immunity to cancer and heart disease.

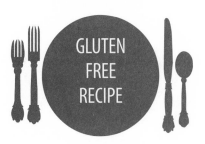

Gluten-Free Rice Bread

DRY INGREDIENTS
1-1/2 cups brown rice flour
1-1/2 cups almond flour
3 teaspoons xanthan gum
1 teaspoon sea salt
1 tablespoon baking powder

WET INGREDIENTS
2 tablespoons maple syrup
2 eggs or egg substitute (see below)
2 tablespoons olive, safflower or canola oil
1 teaspoon apple-cider vinegar
1-1/4 cups water (add 1 tablespoon at a time if too thick)
Egg substitute: 1 tablespoon ground flax seed plus 3 tablespoons water = 1 egg (let set for a few minutes to become gelatinous)

DIRECTIONS
Preheat oven at 350 F. Mix dry ingredients in one bowl and wet ingredients in another. Grease bread pan or line with parchment paper (parchment makes bread easy to lift from baking dish. Put mixture (should be fairly wet but able to lift) into pan and bake for 1 hour.

BENEFITS
Whole brown rice and almond flour supply the critical nutrients copper and manganese to the diet.
Flax seeds supply the anti-inflammatory omega-3 and/or 9 fatty acids.

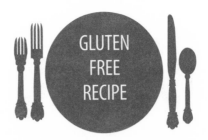

GLUTEN FREE RECIPE

Mediterranean Rice Salad

INGREDIENTS
1-1/2 cups long-grain brown or black rice (forbidden rice)
3 cups cold water
1/2 teaspoon salt
1/4 cup fresh-squeezed lemon juice
1/4 cup extra virgin olive oil
1 tablespoon fresh minced oregano, or 1 teaspoon dried oregano
3 tablespoons fresh minced basil
1 teaspoon salt
1/4 teaspoon black pepper
2 cups spinach leaves, wash, remove stems and chop (To save time you can use prewashed baby spinach)
1/2 cup Kalamata olives, chopped
1/2 cup toasted pine nuts
Optional: 1 garlic clove, mince

DIRECTIONS
Rinse rice in cold water to wash away any debris. Place rice and water in a pot (with lid) and bring rice to a boil, uncovered. When it comes to a boil, lower heat to medium or low and cover. Check once in a while to make sure there is still enough water so rice doesn't burn. You can always add a little water and cover with lid. When rice looks done, turn off heat and let rice steam a bit more; fluff with fork.

DRESSING
Mix lemon juice, olive oil, oregano, basil, salt and pepper in a large bowl. Toss the rice into the dressing. Add in spinach, olives, garlic and pine nuts. Serve.

BENEFITS
Brown rice has more nutrients than white rice.
Spinach is a powerful source of iron and anti-cancer vitamin A.
The herbs are a good source of anti-oxidants.
Pine nuts supply vitamin E and are a powerful source of manganese, part of the anti-cancer SOD enzyme.

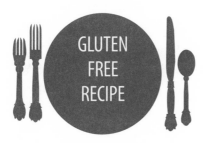

GLUTEN FREE RECIPE

Hummus in the Raw

INGREDIENTS
1 cup chickpeas (soaked 24 hours)
Juice from 2 limes
1 clove garlic, crush
2 tablespoons tahini
1 teaspoon cumin
1 dash of cayenne
1/4 cup fresh chopped parsley
1/2 teaspoon sea salt
1/4 cup water, or more for best consistency

DIRECTIONS
Put lime juice in blender. Rinse soaked chickpeas and pour into blender. Add garlic, cumin, cayenne, salt and parsley. Blend together and add water as needed. Adjust salt to taste. This is delicious on steamed vegetables or fresh veggies.

BENEFITS
Chickpeas are an excellent source of molybdenum (detoxifies the body against alcohol and sulfites).
Sesame seeds are a rich source of the critical element copper.

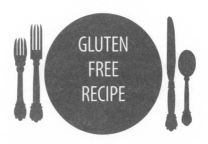

GLUTEN
FREE
RECIPE

Miso Dressing

INGREDIENTS
1/2 cup water
1 tablespoons light-yellow rice soybean miso
1 tablespoon fresh lime or lemon juice
1 tablespoon blackstrap molasses
1 dash of cayenne
1 garlic clove, minced
1 teaspoon toasted sesame oil

DIRECTIONS
Starting with water, blend in miso with a mini-whopper or whisk until totally blended. Add remaining ingredients and blend well. Can be used over salads or steamed vegetables.

BENEFITS
Blackstrap molasses averts copper manganese deficiency in our diets, a deficiency that increases cancer and heart disease rates.

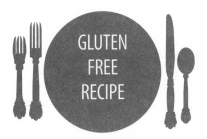

GLUTEN FREE RECIPE

Hemp Seed Crackers

INGREDIENTS

1 cup buckwheat flour
1 cup brown rice flour
1 cup hemp seed meal
1/2 teaspoon sea salt
3 tablespoons unhulled sesame seeds
3 tablespoons dried garlic flakes
1 teaspoon fresh chopped rosemary
4 tablespoons safflower oil
3/4 to 1 cup cold water
Parchment paper, size to fit inside baking sheet
Salt for sprinkling on top

Tip

Use other combinations of herbs like basil, cumin, cayenne or oregano. Experiment with other flours such as rice or oat flour or throw in some raw sunflower seeds. It's best to keep some kind of seed or nut meal in the mix. They are so easy to make. We use safflower oil to bake the crackers because it withstands the high heat.

DIRECTIONS

Preheat oven to 350 F. Mix dry ingredients in a large bowl so you can blend everything well. Add safflower oil and blend with pastry blender until evenly mixed. Add half of the water and mix. By this time you will probably want to start kneading with your hands. Add more water, little by little, and keep kneading until the dough comes together into a cohesive ball. Only use enough water to hold together, not sticky. This only takes a few minutes. Divide dough into even halves. On parchment paper press dough into an oblong shape and start to roll with a rolling pin from the center outward. You also can place a piece of parchment on top of dough before rolling if you prefer, but not necessary. Roll to 1/16-inch thick. Score the dough into squares or desired shape. Prick each square 2 or 3 times with a fork. Sprinkle sesame and sea salt on top and press gently with rolling pin. Transfer parchment sheet of cracker dough to cookie sheet and bake 20 minutes or until golden brown. Turn baking sheet half way through baking time. Roll out second batch while first batch is baking. Let crackers cool before breaking apart. Store in airtight container. Makes about 3 cups of crackers.

BENEFITS

Hemp seeds contain copper and iron and high-quality protein that is easily assimilated.
Safflower oil is a powerful source of anti-cancer omega 9.
Buckwheat is loaded with artery-saving anti-oxidants like rutin.

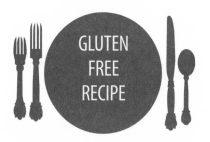

Silver Dollar Buckwheat Pancakes

INGREDIENTS
1 cup buckwheat flour
1 teaspoon sea salt
1 teaspoon baking powder (gluten and aluminum free)
1 tablespoon safflower oil
1-1/4 cups water
3 tablespoons green onion, slice thin

DIRECTIONS
Combine dry ingredients in small bowl. Combine water and oil in measuring cup or other bowl. Stir wet ingredients into flour mixture until smooth. Stir in green onions. Spoon tablespoonfuls of batter onto a lightly greased cast-iron skillet that has been heated. When bubbles appear leaving holes in the pancakes, turn over and brown other side.
To serve, place on plate, salt lightly on top and drizzle on butter or safflower oil. Sour cream is a nice topping also. Or, slather with green olive tapenade for a simple lunch (see tapenade recipe). Makes about a dozen.

BENEFITS
Buckwheat is a rich source of artery-saving anti-oxidants such as rutin.
Safflower oil is a rich source of anti-inflammatory and anti-cancer omega-9.

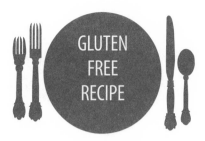

Quinoa Tabbouleh

INGREDIENTS
2 cups cooked and cooled quinoa, (see below for cooking instructions)
1 cup finely chopped parsley
1/2 cup chopped scallions
1 garlic clove, press
2 tablespoons chopped fresh mint
1 tablespoon minced sweet basil
1/2 teaspoon salt (or to taste)
Pinch or 1/8 teaspoon cayenne pepper (or black pepper to taste)
1/2 cup fresh lemon or lime juice
1/4 cup extra virgin olive oil

DIRECTIONS
Rinse quinoa 2 to 3 times. This helps remove some of the slight bitter taste.
For cooking the ratio is 2 parts water to 1 part quinoa. Add water to a kettle and bring water to a boil. Add quinoa and bring back to a boil. Cover and cook over medium heat for 12 minutes or until quinoa has absorbed all the water. Remove from heat. Fluff with fork. Cover to let stand for 15 minutes.

Toss all ingredients together and chill for 1 hour or more before serving.

BENEFITS
Complete protein that is gluten free.
Parsley is a good source of fiber and anti-cancer substances.
Fiber helps colon health.
Olive oil supplies anti-cancer omega-3 fatty acids.

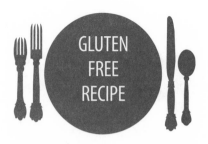

Veggie Burgers

INGREDIENTS
1 cup cooked brown rice
1 cup cooked red lentils
1/2 red onion
3 tablespoons green onion (white part)
3 small organic carrots
2 cups raw mushrooms
3 tablespoons safflower oil
1/8 teaspoon fresh rosemary
1/2 teaspoon dried thyme
1 teaspoon fresh basil
1 large garlic clove
Salt and pepper to taste
Optional: pinch of cayenne

DIRECTIONS
Place carrots and onions in food processor and pulse into small pieces, but not watery mushy. Take out of processor and put in mushrooms. Pulse mushrooms until small pieces. In a pan with 1 tablespoon of oil, brown mushrooms over medium heat. Take out of pan and put aside. In same pan with 1 tablespoon of oil, toss in onion and carrot mixture. Stir, add cover and cook about 5 to 10 minutes. Be sure to uncover and stir now and then. When done, turn off heat. Mix in spices and herbs.
Mix in rice and lentils and shape into burgers by pressing mixture in palm of hand and turning over and pressing more until shape holds together and its flattened as much as possible. Place on a plate, cover and chill for 1/2 hour or longer.
On an oiled skillet, place patties and cook until brown on one side. Turn over to brown other side.

BENEFITS
The combination of rice and lentils allows the burgers to supply a complete protein that is the equivalent of meat.
Whole grains supply more copper and manganese than refined grains.
Spices and herbs supply anti-oxidants.

Bibliography

REFERENCES

chapter one

1. Bisset, Norman Grainger. *Herbal Drugs And Phytopharmaceuticals*. 1 ed. Ann Arbor: CRC Press, 1994.

2. Ravenscroft, A. B. et al. *Daily nutritional intake and serum lipid levels. The Tecumseh study*. American Journal Clinical Nutrition. 1976: 29(12) 1384-1392.

3. O'Dell, B.L. et al. *Mineral deficiencies of milk and congenital malformations in the rat*. Journal of Nutrition. 1961: 73, 151-157.

4. Carlton, W.W. and Henderson, W. *Cardiovascular lesions in experimental copper deficiency in chickens*. Journal of Nutrition. 1963: 81, 200-208.

5. Spiekerman, R.E. et al. *The spectrum of coronary heart disease in a community of 30,000*. Circulation. 1962: 55-57.

6. Berliner, J. *Oral Presentation*. UCLA School Of Public Health, 1989.

7. Steinkühler, C. *Increase of superoxide dismutase activities during differentiation of human K562 cells involves activation by copper*. J Biol Chem. 1991: 266, 24580-24587.

8. Changdong, Yan, et al. *Increased superoxide leads to decreased flow induced dilation in resistance in arteries of MN-SOD deficient mice*. J Physiol Heart Circ Physiology. 2005: 288: H2225-H2231.

9. Qiung, Lu et al. *Superoxide and endothelium dependant constriction to flow in porcine small pulmonary arteries*. British Journal of Pharmacology. 2009: 124(2) 331-336.

10. Didion, Sean et al. *Overexpression of CuZN-SOD prevents lipopolysaccharide induced endothelial dysfunction*. Journal of American Heart Association. 2004: 35(8) p1963-1967.

11. Hill, C.H. et al. *Role of copper in the formation of elastin*. 1967: Fed Proc, 26, 129.

12. Klevay, L. M., Viestenz K. E. *Abnormal cardiograms in rats deficient in copper*. American Journal of Physiology. 1981: 240, H185-H189.

13. Swift, A. et al. *Low prostaglandin concentrations cause cardiac rhythm disturbances. Effect reversed by low levels of copper or chloroquine*. Prostaglandins. 1978: 15 651-657.

14. Klevay L. *Atrial thrombosis, abnormal electrocardiograms and sudden death in mice due to copper deficiency*. Atherosclerosis, Elsevier. 1985: 54(2), 213-224.

15. Klevay L. M. and Forbush, J. *Copper metabolism and the epidemiology of coronary heart disease*. Nutr Rep Int. 1976: 14, 221-228.

16. Mills, C. F. et al. *The preparation of a semi-synthetic diet low in copper for copper-deficiency studies with the rat*. Journal of Food Science. 1960: 11(9) 547-552.

17. Menino, A. R., Damron, W.S. Influence of dietary copper on reproduction of Swiss Webster female mice. Lab Animal Sci. 1986: (2) 164-7.

18. Reiser, S. et al. Indices of copper status in humans consuming a typical American diet. Am J. Clin Nutr. 1985: 42, 242-251.

19. Casey, C. E., et al. *Copper, manganese, zinc in New Zealanders*. Biol. Trace Element research. 1982: 4:105-115.

20. Klevay L. M. *Deliberations on dietary recommendations about copper*. RDA workshops, USDA, Grand Forks, N. D., September 10-12. 1995: p24238. (Downloaded from www.Jn.nutrition.org on 11.13, 2010.)

21. Jariwalla, R. J. *Microcompetition and the origin of cancer*. European Journal of Cancer. 2005: 4(1) 15-19.

22. Polansky, H. *Microcompetition with foreign DNA and the origin of chronic disease.* Center for the Biology of Chronic Disease, 3159 S. Winston Road, Rochester NY 14623.

23. Sohrenson, P. and Autor, A.P., ed. *Pathology of Oxygen,* Chapter 13, Academic Press, New York, 1982.

24. Sahu, S. K. *Effects of dexamethasone on neuroblastoma cell differentiation.* Ann Arbor: University Microfilms International, 1979. Abstract in reference 23.

25. Oberley, L. *Role of SOD in Cancer, A Review (see last paragraph, injection of SOD into tumors).* Cancer Research. 1979: 39, 1147.

26. Morishige, Fukumi, et al. *J Nutr Growth and Cancer. 1983:* 1, 67. See also F. Morishige, et al. *The role of vitamin C in tumor therapy (Human) page 405-406 in Vitamins and cancer: human cancer prevention by vitamins and micronutrients.* Frank L. Meyskens Jr., ed. New Jersey: Humana Press, Inc., 1986.

27. Werts, E. D., Gould, M. N. *Relationship between cellular superoxide dismutase and susceptibility to chemically induced cancer in the rat mammary gland.* Carcinogenesis, Oxford University Press. 1986: 7(7) 1197-1201.

28. List of Cruciferous vegetables. *http://en.wikipedia.org/wiki/Cruciferous_vegetables.*

29. Dudai, N., Weinstein, Y., Krup, M., Rabinski, T. and Ofir, R. *Citral is a new inducer of caspase-3 in tumor cell lines.* Planta Medica. 2005: 71: 484-488.

30. Carter, J. P. *Hypothesis: Dietary management may improve survival from nutrionally linked cancers.* Journal of American College of Nutrition. 1993: 12(2), 209-206.

31. Caughey, G. E . *The effect on human tumor necros is factor and interleukin 1ß production of diets enriched -3 fatty acids from vegetable or fish oils.* American Journal of Clinical Nutrition. 1996: 63, 116-122.

32. Smith, R. L. et al. *In vitro stimulation, of articular chondrocyte mRNA and extracellular matrix synthesis, by hydrostatic pressure.* Journal of Orthopaedic Res. 14(1) 53-60, 1996.

33. Murray, J. et al. *Prevalence of celiac disease in the United States.* Arch. Int. Med. 2003: 163, 286-292.

chapter two

34. Weindruch, R. et, al. *The retardation of aging and disease by dietary restriction.* Springfield: Charles C. Thomas, 1988.

35. Berg, T. F. et al. *Acute toxicity of ganciclovir, effect of dietary restriction and chronobiology.* Food Chem Toxicol. 1994: 32(1) 45-50.

36. Heydori, A. R. et al. *Expression of heat shock protein 70 is altered by age and diet at the level of transcription.* Mol and Cell Biology. 1993: 13(5) 2909-29018.

37. Merry, B. J. *Molecular mechanisms linking calorie restriction and longevity.* Int J Biol Cell Biol. 2002: 34, 1340-1354.

38. Wilcox, B. J. et al. *Caloric restriction the traditional Okinawan diet, and healthy aging.* Ann, New York: Acad Sci. 2007: 1114, 434 455.

39. Roth, G. S. et al. *Biomarkers of caloric restriction may predict longevity in humans.* New York: Science. 2002: 297(5582) 81.

40. Kalimi, M. et al. *DHEA, Biochemical Physiological and Clinical Aspects.* New York: Walter de Guyter Publishing, 1999.

41. Harrison, D. E. et al. *Effects of food restriction on aging.* USA: Proc Natl Acad Science. 1984: 81, 1835-1838.

42. Eaton, B. S., Cordain, L. *Evolutionary aspects of diet, old genes, new fuels.* Nutrition and Fitness. Evolutionary health, Childrens health. Sinopoulos, A. P. (ed.) Basel Karger. 1997: 81, 26-37.

43. Anderson, J. W. et al. *Health benefits and practical aspects of high fiber diets.* American Journal of Clinical Nutrition. 1994: 59, 1242-1247.

44. Anderson, J. W. et al. *Treatment of diabetes with high fiber diet.* CRC Handbook Of Dietary Fiber On Human Nutrition. 1993: 443-70, Spiller, G. A. ed. Boca Raton: CRC Press.

45 . Kalant, N., Stewart, J. *Effect of diet restriction on glucose metabolism and insulin responsiveness in aging rats.* Mech. Ageing Dev. 1988: 46(1-3) 89-104.

46. Lane, M. A., Ingram, D. K. *Calorie restriction in non-human primates.* Toxicol Sci. 1999: 52(2) 41-48.

47. Lane, M. A., Ingram, D. K. *Calorie restriction in non human primates.* Ann, New York: Acad Sci. 2001: 928 287-295.

48. Yu, B. P. *Aging and oxidative stress modulation by dietary restriction.* Free Radic Biol Med. 1996: 21(5) 651-668.

49. Yu, B. P. Chung. HY. *Stress resistance by caloric restriction for longevity.* New York: Acad Sc. 2001: 928 39-47.

50. Dubey, A. et al. *Effect of age and caloric intake on protein oxidations in different brain regions of the mouse.* Arch Biochem. 1996: 333 189-197.

51. Lin, Y. J., Seroude, L. *Extended life span and stress resistance in the drosophila mutant Methuselah.* Science. 1998: 282(5390), 943-946.

52. Armeni, T. et al. *Studies of the life prolonging effect of food restriction, glutathione and glyoxylase enzymes in the liver.* Mech Aging Dev. 1998: 101(1-2), 101-110.

53. Weindruch, R. *The Retardation of Aging and Disease By Dietary Restriction.* Charles C Thomas, Publisher, Springfield IL 1988.

54. Kritchevsky D. Dietary fat versus caloric content in initiation and promotion of DMBA induced mammary tumours in rats. Cancer Res. 198: 44(8) 3174-3177.

55. Schütz, B. et al. *Production of the tissue inhibitor of metalloproteinase-2 (TIMP-2) and evaluation of its potential as anti-aging active.* Int J Cosm Sci. 2006: 28(1), 69-69.

56. Wu, A. et al. *Soy intake and risk of breast cancer in Asian Americans* American Journal of Clinical Nutrition. 1998: 68(6) 51437-51443.

57. Bergamini, E. et al. *The anti-aging effects of calorie restriction may involve stimulation of macroautophagy and lysosomal degradation.* Biomed & Pharmacotherapy. 2003: 57(506) 203-208. See also Stevens, A., Lowe, J. *Pathology.* London, England: Mosby, 2000.

58. Mortimer, G. E. et al. *Intracellular protein catabolism and its control during nutrient deprivation and supply.* Annu Rev. Nutr. 1987: 7, 534-64.

chapter four

59. Rashimi, Sinha. P*an-fried meat containing high levels of polycyclic aromatic hydrocarbons induces cytochrome P4501A2 activity in humans.* Cancer research.1994: 54, 6154-6159.

60. Woessner, Warren W., Evehjem, C. A., and Schuette, Henry A., *The determination of ascorbic acid in commercial milks.* Journal of Nutrition. December, 1939: 18,6:619-626.

61. McAfee, Mark. *Letter to the Colorado Department Of Public Health.* Denver, Colorado, May 19, 2004. *www.realmilk.com2010.*

chapter six

62. Dr. Richard Schulze. *Cleanse and heal your body with Dr Schulze's 5 day bowel detox.* Natural Healing Publications, 2007.

chapter seven

63. Sanchez, Albert et al. *Role of sugars in human neutrophilic phagocytosis.* American Journal of Clinical Nutrition. 1973: 26, 1180-1184.

64. Nancy Appleton. *146 reasons why sugar is ruining your health.* www.rheumatic.org/sugar. htm. 146 references included.

chapter nine

65. Ferenczi, Alexander. Austr. Int Clin Rev. July, 1986.

66. Kapadia, G. J. et al. *Chemoprevention of DMBA-induced UV-B promoted, NOR-1-induced TPA promoted skin carcinogenesis, and DEN-induced phenobarbital promoted liver tumors in mice by extract of beetroot.* Pharmacol Res. Feb. 2003: 47(2):141-8.

67. Halverson, B. L. et al. *A Systematic Screening of Total Antioxidants in Dietary Plants.* The Journal of Nutrition. 2002: 132(3):461-71.

68. Khahn, Alam et al. *Cinnamon Improves Glucose and Lipids of People With Type 2 Diabetes.* Diabetes Care. December, 2003: vol. 26 no. 12 3215-3218.

69. Green, K. N. et al. *"Dietary docosahexaenoic acid and docosapentaenoic acid ameliorate amyloid- and tau pathology via a mechanism involving presenilin 1 levels".* J Neuroscience. 2007: 27 (16): 4385–4395.

70. Peet, M. and Horrobin, D. F. *A dose-ranging study of the effects of ethyl-eicosapentaenoate in patients with ongoing depression despite apparently adequate treatment with standard drugs.* Archives of General Psychiatry. October, 2002: Vol. 59, pp. 913-19.

71. Nagakura T. *Dietary supplementation with fish oil rich in omega-3 polyunsaturated fatty acids in children with bronchial asthma.* Eur Respir Journal. 2000: 16:861-865.

72. Casey, T.R. and Bamforth, C.W. "Silicon in Beer and Brewing." *Journal of the Science of Food and Agriculture.* Published Online: February 8, 2010 (DOI: 10.1002/JSFA.3884). Print Issue Date: February 2010.

73. Vinson, J. et al. *Dried Fruits: Excellent in Vitro and in Vivo Antioxidants.* Journal of the American College of Nutrition. 2005: Vol. 24, No. 1, 44-50.

74. Ernst, E. and Pittler, M. H. *Efficacy of ginger for nausea and vomiting: a systematic review of randomized clinical trials.* British Journal of Anaesthesia. 2000: Vol 84, Issue 3, 367-371.

75. Rhode, J. M. et al. *Ginger induces apoptosis and autophagocytosis in ovarian cancer cells.* Abstract #4510, presented April 4, 2006 at the 97th AACR Annual Meeting, April 1-5, 2006, Washington, DC, 2006.

76. Diouf, A. et al. *Dietary intake of fluorine through tea prepared by the traditional method.* Senegal Dakar Med. 1994: 39(2):227-30. Article in French with English abstract.

77. Osburn, Lynn. *Hemp Line Journal.* July-August, 1992: pp.14-15, Vol. I No. 1

78. Percival, Susan S. *Neoplastic Transformation of BALB/3T3 Cells and Cell Cycle of HL-60 Cells are Inhibited by Mango (Mangifera indica L.) Juice and Mango Juice Extracts.* Jour Nutr. 2006: 136:1300-1304,

79. Hirazumi, A. et al. *Anticancer activity of Morinda citrifolia (Noni) on intraperitoneally implanted lewis lung carcinoma in syngeneic mice.* Proc Western Pharmacog. Soc. 1994: 37: 145-146.

80. Sen, C. K., Khanna, S., Roy, S. *"Tocotrienols: Vitamin E beyond tocopherols".* Life Sciences. 2006: 78 (18): 2088–98.

81. Weng-Yew, W. et al. *"Suppression of tumor growth by palm tocotrienols via the attenuation of angiogenesis".* Nutrition and Cancer. 2009: 61 (3): 367–73.

82. Wali, V. B., Bachawal, S. V., Sylvester, P. W. *"Combined treatment of gamma-tocotrienol with statins induce mammary tumor cell cycle arrest in G1."* Experimental Biology and Medicine. 2009: 234 (6): 639–50.

83. Joubert, Elizabeth et al. *Superoxide anion and a, a-diphenyl-β-picrylhydrazyl radical scavenging capacity of rooibos (Aspalathus linearis) aqueous extracts, crude phenolic fractions, tannin and flavonoids.* Food Research International. March 2004: Volume 37, Issue 2, pages 133-138.

84. Marnewick, J. *Rooibos and heart disease, unpublished studies, Rooibos Science Café.* Cape Town: MTN Scien Centre, 26 November, 2008.

85. Fajardo-Lira, C. *Effect of brewing method on anti-oxidant activity of rooibos tea.* 2005 IFT Annual Meeting, July 15 to 20, New Orleans, Louisiana. Presentation 18E-13.

86. Menendez, J. A. et al. *Dietary fatty acids regulate the activation status of Her-2/neu (c-erb B-2) oncogene in breast cancer cells.* Annals Oncology. 2004: 15, page 1719-1723.

87. Meyers, Katherine J. et al. *Anti-oxidant and Anti-proliferative Activities of Strawberries.* J. Agric. Food Chem. 2003: 51 (23), pp 6887–6892.

88. Harris, W. S. et al. *Comparison of the effects of fish and fish-oil capsules on the omega–3 fatty acid content of blood cells and plasma phospholipids.* American Journal of Clinical Nutrition. December 2007: Vol. 86, No. 6, 1621-1625.

89. Stone, Irwin. *The Healing Factor "Vitamin C" Against Disease.* New York: Grosset & Dunlap, 1972: page 153, 1978 printing.

90. Ah-Ng, Tony Kong, et al. *Combined Inhibitory Effects of Curcumin and Phenethyl Isothiocyanate on the Growth of Human PC-3 Prostate Xenografts in Immunodeficient Mice.* Cancer Research. January 15, 2006: 66, 613-621.

91. Gann, Peter H. et al. *Lower Prostate Cancer Risk in Men with Elevated Plasma Lycopene Levels.* Cancer Research. March 1, 1999: 59, 1225-1230.

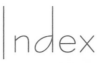

Index

REFERENCES

Acai berry, freeze-dried - 127

Acerola cherries - 52, 84, 113, 125, 127

Acetylenics - 137

Advil - 34, 36

ALA - 37-42, 137, 159

Alcohol - 103, 109, 120, 122, 131, 137, 147, 157

Aldehyde - 31, 59, 130, 136, 146

Almonds - 17, 18, 52, 73, 83, 125, 126, 131, 154

Aloe Vera- 107, 109

Alzheimer's Disease- 59, 131-134

Amines- 90, 92, 160

Amylase- 90

Anethole - 141

Anthocyanidins - 129

Anthocyanins - 129, 130, 131, 133, 135, 146, 152, 155, 164

Anti-inflammatories - 31, 118, 136

Antibiotics - 68, 79, 97, 103, 110, 111, 144

Antivirals - 147

Apples - 16, 17, 88, 107, 122, 126, 128, 152, 164

Apricots - 126, 128

Arachidonic Acid - 35, 38, 39, 138

Arginine - 92, 123

Arrowroot - 50, 51

Arsenic - 68, 79, 80

Aromatase - 149

Arthritis - 31-38, 40-45, 48, 49, 54, 55, 76, 81, 112, 114, 123, 128, 132, 151, 159, 162, 166

Aspartame - 104

Astaxanthin - 42

Atrial Fibrillation - 160

Atrial Thrombosis - 75

Avenacosides - 150

Avocado - 82, 101, 125, 126, 128

Aztecs - 137

Barbecuing - 84, 92, 141

Barley - 48-50, 85, 126, 129, 139

Beans, dried - 16, 17, 31, 71, 82-85, 89, 92, 93, 124, 126, 131

Beans, black - 108, 126, 132

Beef - 16, 29, 40, 43, 60, 67, 71-76, 82-86, 93, 94, 102, 124, 126, 131, 132

Beer - 49, 74, 130, 139

Bell peppers - 52, 82, 84, 108, 126, 132

Betaine - 142

Betacyanin - 132

Blackcurrants - 126, 132

Blueberries - 84, 126, 129, 133, 137

Bone marrow - 26, 109

Borscht - 93, 132

Bowel84, 105-109, 114, 132, 145, 152, 155, 164, 166

Bran - 30, 85, 87, 137, 166

Bran, Oat - 52, 151

Bran, Rice - 85, 157

Brazil nuts - 18, 30, 52, 86, 91, 126, 133

Broccoli - 16, 29, 70, 74, 82, 84, 88, 91, 93, 108, 126, 133, 139, 148

Buckwheat - 43, 49, 51, 87, 126, 133, 137, 163

Bulgur wheat - 126, 134

Brussels sprouts - 84, 91, 126, 133, 139, 148

Breast Cancer - 20, 22, 25, 59, 62, 88, 134, 139, 145, 148, 150, 156, 158, 165

Buffalo - 32, 78

Cabbage - 29, 74, 84, 91, 93, 124, 133, 134, 139, 146, 148

Caffiec Acid - 128, 139

Caffeine - 86, 159

Cantaloupe - 126, 165, 164

Caloric Restriction - 56, 63

Cane Sugar - 18, 48, 55, 59, 115

Carminative - 142

Carnosine - 60, 84, 131,

Carrots - 17, 50, 70, 74, 82, 84, 88, 108, 118, 126, 128, 135, 156

Cartilage - 31, 43, 45, 47, 61, 129, 139

Casein - 55, 71

Cashews - 17, 43, 83, 126, 135

Cataracts - 115, 129, 143, 146, 148

Celebrex - 36

Celery - 70, 88, 126, 128, 135

Celiac Disease - 45-52, 89, 104

Cheetos - 54

Cherries - 84, 113, 126, 127, 136

Chia seed (salba) - 43, 52, 67, 83, 85, 126, 136

Chickpeas - 51, 126, 137, 145

Chocolate - 16, 52, 74, 83, 86, 126, 140

Chondroitin Sulfate - 30, 43, 47

Chymopapain - 153

Cinnamon (spice) - 115, 126, 137, 163

Clams - 15, 47, 126, 138

Cloves (spice) - 84, 126, 138, 141, 165

Cod - 52, 73, 74, 126, 138, 160

Coenzyme Q10 - 42

Collagen - 13, 31, 38, 47, 61, 77, 99, 112, 127, 129

Collard greens - 29, 84, 91, 93, 126, 139

Colorectal Cancer - 105

Constipation - 49, 106-108, 120, 134, 143, 154, 160

Coumarins - 136

COX Enzymes - 35, 38, 39, 136, 164

Cranberries - 126, 138

Crohn's Disease - 165

CRON - 56-60

Cruciferous vegetables - 29, 30, 84, 85, 93, 94, 107, 126, 131-139, 165

Cryptoxanthin - 132, 153

Cucumber - 82, 126, 139, 153

Curcumin - 165

Cytokines - 34, 137

Cyperone - 143

Cyanidin - 155

Cystic Fibrosis - 165

Cyclo-Oxygenases - 35, 38, 164

Cysteine - 62

Dates - 85, 115, 126, 140

Dehydration - 119, 120, 123

Depression - 49, 74, 114, 138, 161

DHA - 37, 40-42, 159

Diabetes - 38, 49, 55, 58, 66, 76, 89,
    90, 98, 114, 139, 142

Diarrhea - 47, 61, 106, 108, 112, 120,
    154

Diverticulitis - 106, 128, 134, 138

DNA - 30, 92, 133, 143, 146, 152

Docosapentaenoic Acid - 37

Dramamine - 142

Eicosapentenoic Acid - 37, 42, 159

Ellagitannins - 155, 163

Emphysema - 114, 132, 135, 163

EPA - 36, 39-42, 49, 159, 165

Estrogen - 21, 62, 149

Excedrin - 36

Exercise - 122

Fatigue - 48, 104, 120

Fibromyalgia - 104

Figs - 126, 140, 141, 155

Fish Oil - 40-43, 159, 165

Flavonoids - 113, 122, 134, 144, 147,
    153, 157

Flaxseed - 39-41, 83, 126, 136, 140,
    141, 151, 159

Fluoride - 83, 121, 143, 158, 161

Gamma-linoleic Acid - 38, 159

Garlic - 91, 108, 126, 141, 148, 152

Ginger - 47, 126, 142, 153

Grapefruit - 84, 126, 143

Green tea - 86, 126, 143, 158

Glaucoma - 129

Gliadin - 48, 89

Globulin - 85, 144, 145, 149

Glucosamine - 31, 43, 44, 46-48

Glucose - 54, 58, 59-65, 69, 82, 101,
    104, 113-115, 123, 132, 134, 154

Glucosinolates - 93, 132, 160

Glutathione - 29, 58, 133, 153, 158,
    164

Glutamin - 123, 124

Gluten - 48-51, 82, 104, 134, 155

Glycation - 58, 64, 93, 101, 104, 131

Goitrogens - 94, 91, 161

Halibut - 30, 126, 144, 153

Halal Foods - 103

HDL - 13, 77

Hemorrhoids - 108, 114, 129

Hemp seeds - 126, 144

Hemp seed oil - 83, 86, 126, 145, 151

Herring - 88, 126, 145

Heterocyclic Aromatic - 90, 92

HGH - 122-124

Homogenization - 95, 99

Hormones - 34, 38, 97, 103, 149, 150

Hummus - 52, 62, 65, 82, 86, 108, 126,
    132, 134, 145

Hydrocarbons - 29

Hydrochloric Acid - 101, 134

Hydrogen Peroxide - 29, 112, 152

Hydrogenated Oil - 23, 104, 140

Hyperbaric Therapy - 119, 124

Ibuprofen - 36, 39

Infectious Disease - 54, 112, 114

Insomnia - 142

Insulin - 57-59, 79, 112, 122

Iodine - 54, 78, 91, 94, 148, 161, 165

Irradiation - 89

Isocyanates - 94

Kale - 29, 50, 85, 91, 93, 126, 128, 146

Kidney - 34, 66, 101, 114, 120, 138,
    142

Kidney beans - 71

Kidney stones - 139

Kiwi fruit - 53, 113, 126, 146

Kohlrabi - 29, 84, 91, 93, 139

Kosher Foods - 103

Krill Oil - 40, 42

Lactobacilli - 97

Lactose - 54, 96, 97, 148

L- Carnosine - 131

LDL - 13, 77

Lemongrass - 30

Lentils - 71, 85, 126, 147

Lentinan - 148

L-ergothionine - 148

Ligaments - 31, 33, 44, 46, 61, 104,
    112, 139

Limonene - 143

Linoleic Acid - 159

Lipase - 90, 96, 147

Liver - 34, 39, 63, 66, 112, 114, 120,
    128, 142, 148, 158, 164

Lutein - 128, 146

Lycopene - 128, 132, 143, 153, 166

Lycophene - 42, 102

Macroautophagy - 79

Magnesium - 36, 39, 79, 116, 120, 144

Maple Syrup - 18, 86, 115, 126, 147,
    158

Margarine - 16, 38

Matrix Metalloproteinase - 62

Melatonin - 136

Mercury - 15, 41, 153, 165

Methyl sulfonyl methane - 44

Millet - 48, 50, 91

Monsosodium Glutamate - 54

MRI - 32, 45

Molybdenum - 130, 137, 146, 147,
    154

Morning Sickness - 142

Motion Sickness - 142

Mucous - 50, 96

Mucous membranes - 50, 118, 156

Mushrooms - 52, 74, 126, 148, 152

Mustard - 60, 63, 94, 126, 148

Mustard greens - 29, 84, 91, 126,
    139, 148

Myrosinase - 94

Neuroblastoma - 25

NSAIDS - 32, 34, 37, 39, 43, 46, 49

Nettle - 126, 149

Noni juice - 126, 149

Oat bran - 52, 126, 151, 157

Oats - 48, 73, 85, 126, 130, 149

Obesity - 53, 55, 61, 67, 70, 91, 98,
    115, 144, 161

Olive oil - 37, 40, 44, 52, 65, 83, 86,
    126, 145, 151, 153, 156, 159

Omega-3 - 31, 34, 36-47, 52, 62, 67,
    74, 77, 79, 83, 101, 119, 159,
    163, 165

ORAC - 42, 92, 127

Oranges - 84, 122, 126, 152

Oregano - 126, 152

Oregon Grape - 108

Organosulfur - 139, 141

Osteoporosis - 47, 49, 96, 114

Ovaries - 162

Oysters - 15-18, 27, 29, 31, 47, 83, 95, 103, 126, 153

Palm oil - 50, 126, 130, 156, 163

Papain - 153

Papaya - 52, 84, 113, 126, 153

Parsley - 124, 126, 134, 154, 162

Pasteurization - 95, 147

PCB's - 40, 144

Pecans - 126, 154

Pepper, black - 154

Peptic ulcers - 129

Phagocytes - 111

Phosphatase - 96

Phthalides - 135

Physalin - 142

Phytosterol - 162

Pinto beans - 126, 154

Plantago - 108

Plantar Fasciitis - 46

Plaque - 11-13, 83, 127, 134, 139, 141

Plums - 141, 155, 126

Polycyclic aromatic - 29, 113

Polyphenols - 134

Polyps - 106, 133, 165

Prolotherapy - 47

Prostate - 21, 143, 150

Prostate cancer - 21, 31, 132, 163, 165

Prostaglandins - 34, 38

Protease - 90, 92, 130, 131

Proxeronine - 149

Psoriasis - 142

Quinoa - 49, 50, 82, 126, 155

Raspberries - 126, 155

Resveratrol - 60, 122, 157

Rooibos tea - 126, 145, 158, 159

Rosemary - 126, 158

Rutin - 134

Rye - 48, 50

Safflower oil - 37, 40, 43, 52, 83, 151, 159

Salmon Oil - 40

Salmon - 30, 40, 43, 52, 82, 126, 159

Sardines - 52, 83, 126

Sauerkraut - 29, 84, 94, 126, 134, 148, 160

Scallops - 126, 153, 160

Schizophrenia - 49

Scurvy - 96, 144

Seal oil - 42

Seaweed - 40, 126, 161

Secretagogue - 124

Senna - 109

Sesame seed - 16, 27, 52, 83, 126, 162

SHBG - 149

Silicon - 130

Silymarin - 128

Solavetivone - 143

Spelt - 48, 50

Squash - 50, 65, 74, 84, 126, 135, 163

Stevia - 86, 115

Strawberries - 52, 84, 91, 126, 163

Stomach - 34-39, 49, 75, 91, 101, 119

Sucrose - 55, 59, 104

Sunflower seeds - 93, 156, 163

Spirulina - 140

Sulfite - 130, 146

Sunflower oil - 163

Sweet potatoes - 50, 84, 91, 126, 164

Swiss chard - 126, 164

Testosterone - 21, 85, 149-151

Theobromine - 140

Thromboxane A2 - 137

Thyroid - 23, 30, 91, 94

TIMPS - 62

Tocopherols - 130, 156, 163

Tocotrienols - 130, 156

TSH - 91

Tuberculosis - 26, 95, 111

Turkey - 46, 74, 82, 84, 93, 95, 102

Turmeric - 126, 130, 148, 165

Tumors - 20, 24, 25, 30, 59, 142

Tuna - 164

Tylenol - 36

Tyrosine - 161

Umami - 54

Uterus - 161

Varicose veins - 114, 129

Vegan - 65, 70, 71, 74, 76, 78

Ventricular Repolarization - 161

Vitamin B3 - 112

Vitamin B6 - 141

Vitamin B12 - 131, 138, 146, 152, 160

Vodka - 49

Watercress - 84, 93, 94, 126, 166

Watermelon - 126, 166

Wine - 21, 60, 74, 82, 86, 122, 126, 157

Whiskey - 49

White blood cells - 12, 26, 111-113, 118

Xeronine - 149

Yogurt - 85, 115, 126, 167

Yucca - 126

Zeaxanthin - 146

Zinc - 14, 15, 18, 24, 39, 50, 68, 78

Tables

capacity

ENGLISH TO METRIC

1/5 teaspoon = 1 milliliter
1 teaspoon = 5 milliliters
1 tablespoon = 15 milliliters = 1/2 fluid
ounce
2 tablespoons = 1 fluid ounce
1/5 cup = 50 milliliters
1 cup = 8 ounces or 240 milliliters or
240 grams of water
2 cups (1 pint) = 16 ounces or 470
milliliters
4 cups (1 quart) = .95 liter
4 quarts (1 gal.) = 3.8 liters

METRIC TO ENGLISH

1 milliter = 1/5 teaspoon
5 milliters = 1 teaspoon
15 milliters = 1 tablespoon
29.6 milliters l = 1 fluid oz.
100 milliters = 3.4 fluid oz.
240 milliters = 1 cup
1 liter = 34 fluid ounces
1 liter = 4.2 cups
1 liter = 2.1 pints
1 liter = 1.06 quarts
1 liter = .26 gallon

weight

LIQUID

1 fluid ounce = 30 milliters
1 fluid ounce = 28 grams
1 pound = 454 grams

DRY

1 gram = .035 ounce
28.4 grams = 1 ounce weight
100 grams = 3.5 ounces weight
500 grams = 1.10 pounds
1 kilogram = 2.205 pounds
1 kilogram = 35 oz.

cooking

16 tablesppns = 1 cup
12 tablespoons = 3/4 cup
10 tablespoons + 2 teaspoons = 2/3
cup
8 tablespoons = 1/2 cup
6 tablespoons = 3/8 cup
5 tablespoons + 1 teaspoon = 1/3 cup
4 tablespoons = 1/4 cup
2 tablespoons = 1/8 cup
2 tablespoons + 2 teaspoons = 1/6 cup
1 tablespoon = 1/16 cup
2 cups = 1 pint
2 pints = 1 quart
3 teaspoons = 1 tablespoon
48 teaspoons = 1 cup

nutritional

One milligram is 1,000 micrograms.
(Selenium, Iodine) One gram is
1,000 milligrams
1 ppm or part per million is 1 milligram
per kilogram or 1 milligram per
quart of water or 1 milligram per
2.2 pounds
1 milligram of natural vitamin E is 2 IU
of vitamin E.
500 milligrams of vitamin C is 0.5 grams
of vitamin C. 2 of these are 1,000
milligrams of C.
1,000 milligrams of vitamin C is 1 gram
of vitamin C
2,000 milligrams of vitamin C is 2 grams
of vitamin C

Metric Table

weight (or mass)

IMPERIAL UNIT	METRIC UNIT	METRIC UNIT	IMPERIAL UNIT
Ounce	28.35 grams	**0.035 ounces**	Gram
Pound	0.45 kilograms	**2.21 pounds**	Kilogram
UK ton (2240 pounds)	1.02 metric tons	**0.98 UK tons**	UK Metric ton (1000kg)
US ton (2000 pounds)	0.91 tons	**US Metric ton (1000kg)**	1.10 US tons

volume

IMPERIAL UNIT	METRIC UNIT	METRIC UNIT	IMPERIAL UNIT
Teaspoon (UK)	5.92 milliliters	**Milliliters**	0.17 teaspoons (UK)
Teaspoon (US)	4.93 milliliters	**Milliliters**	0.20 teaspoons (US)
Tablespoon (UK)	17.76 milliliters	**10 milliliters**	0.56 tablespoons (UK)
Tablespoon (US)	14.79 milliliters	**10 milliliters**	0.68 tablespoons (US)
Fluid ounce (UK)	28.41 milliliters	**100 milliliters**	3.52 fluid ounces (UK)
Fluid ounce (US)	29.57 milliliters	**100 milliliters**	3.38 fluid ounces (US)
Pint (UK)	0.57 liters	**Liter**	1.76 pints (UK)
Pint (US)	0.47 liters	**Liter**	2.11 pints (US)
Quart (UK)	1.14 liters	**Liter**	0.88 quarts (UK)
Quart (US)	0.95 liters	**Liter**	1.06 quarts (US)
Gallon (UK)	4.55 liters	**Liter**	0.22 gallon (UK)
Gallon (US)	3.79 liters	**Liter**	0.26 gallon (US)

temperature

IMPERIAL UNIT	METRIC UNIT
C = (F - 32) ÷ 1.8	For example: (68 F - 32) ÷ 1.8 = (36) ÷ 1.8 = 20 C
F = (C x 1.8) + 32	For example: (20 C x 1.8) + 32 = (36) + 32 = 68 F

Metric Conversion Chart

temperature

TO CALCULATE	MULTIPLY	BY
Ounces into grams	28	Number of ounces
Grams into ounces	0.035	Number of grams
Pounds into kilograms	0.45	Number of pounds
Kilograms into pounds	2.2	Number of kilograms
Teaspoons into milliliters	5	Number of teaspoons
Tablespoons into milliliters	15	Number of tablespoons
Fluid ounces into milliliters	30	Number of fluid ounces
Milliliters into fluid ounces	0.034	Number of milliliters
Cups into liters	0.24	Number of cups
Pints into liters	0.47	Number of pints
Quarts into liters	0.95	Number of quarts

General Slow Cooker Tips

OVEN TIME	SLOW COOKER HIGH High setting: 300°F (149°C)	SLOW COOKER LOW Low Setting: 200°f (93.3°c)
5 to 30 minutes	1½ to 2½ hours	4 to 6 hours
35 to 45 minutes	2 to 3 hours	6 to 8 hours
50 minutes to 3 hours	4 to 5 hours	8 to 18 hours
FOOD	SLOW COOKER HIGH	SLOW COOKER LOW
Pot Roast	4 to 5 hours	8 to 12 hours
Stew	5 to 6 hours	10 to 12 hours
Ribs	5 to 6 hours	8 to 9 hours
Swiss Steak	5 to 6 hours	8 to 9 hours
Casserole	2 to 4 hours	4 to 9 hours
Rice	2 to 3 hours	5 to 9 hours
Meatloaf	3 to 4 hours	8 to 10 hours
Chicken	3 to 4 hours	7 to 10 hours
Vegetables in Liquid	1 to 3 hours	2 to 4 hours
Baked Potato	2 to 4 hours	8 to 10 hours

Liquid and Dry ingredient conversion chart

BEGINNING BUSHEL MEASUREMENT	Dry	Liquid	Drops	Teaspoon	Tablesppon	Fluid ounce	Cup	Pint	Quart	Peck
1 pinch	X			1/8						
Dash	X	X	3	1/4						
1 teaspoon	X	X	60	1	1/3	1/6				
3 teaspoons	X	X		3	1	1/2				
1 tablespoon	X	X		3	1	1/2				
2 tablespoons	X	X		6	2	1	1/8			
4 tablespoons	X	X		12	4	2	1/4			
5-1/3 tablespoons	X	X		16	5-1/3		1/3			
1 fluid ounce		X		6	2	1	1/8			
1 shot (jigger)		X				1 1/2				
1 gill		X				4				
1 cup	X	X		48	16	8	1	1/2		
2 cups	X	X		96	32	16	2			
4 cups	X	X			64	32	4	1		
16 cups	X	X				128	16		4	
1 fifth (bottle)		X								
1 pint		X		96	32	16	2	1		
1 quart		X		192	64	128	16	8		
1 gallon		X		768						
8 quarts	X									1

Glossary

ALA - Stands for Alpha- linolenic acid and is an omega-3 fatty acid that occurs in vegetable oils.

Alpha- Linolenic Acid - A compound found in vegetable oils such as flax seed and hemp seed oil. The body can convert this to omega-3 fatty acids.

Aldehyde - A toxic substance made from alcohol in the body. Alcohol in itself is not toxic, but the aldehyde is what causes the affects seen from consumption of alcohol. Recovery occurs when the body converts aldehyde to acetic acid also know as vinegar.

Amylase - An enzyme in the saliva and digestive system that digests starch by turning it into glucose.

Anthocyanins and Anthocyanidins - They are flavonoids that give the blue red or purple color to plants and fruits, and they are similar except that anthocyanins include a glucose molecules. Found in good quantity in such foods as black raspberry that has found to reduce cancer of the rat esophagus and colon.

Anti-Gliadin test - A test for celiac disease. The test is for anti-gliadin anti-bodies which are made in the body in response to an allergic reaction to gluten. A value of around 3 is regarded as normal, a value of 200 is regarded as a severe reaction to gluten in the diet.

Arginine - A compound derived by the body from the protein we eat. It is one of the several amino-acids that are the building blocks of protein. The body needs it to make human growth hormone (HGH), which declines as we age and is considered to be one of the causes of aging when lacking in the body.

Arachidonic Acid - A substance occurring in meat and dairy. The body can also make it from Omega-6 fatty acids. The body uses this to make "series 2 prostaglandins" which promote inflammation in the body. Excess inflammation is associated with cancer, arthritis and heart disease.

Aromatase - An enzyme, that converts testosterone into estrogen. In older men this can cause low testosterone levels which are associated with aging.

Astaxanthin - A red substance found in salmon, lobster, shrimp and krill. They get it from algae. It is a powerful anti-oxidant and present in krill oil. It is a carotenoid like vitamin A. It is approved as a food coloring and is natural.

Atrial Fibrillation - This is a lack of strong heart beat in the upper or atrial chambers of the heart. The occurrence increase with old age and it can result in an irregular heart beat.

Atrial Thrombosis - The interruption of blood flow in the arteries, due to a clot and or narrowing of arteries. Interruption of blood flow to the heart can cause a heart attack and interruption of blood flow t the brain can cause a stroke.

Avenocosides - Substances in oats that stimulate the production of testosterone in men and woman. Lower levels of testosterone are associated with aging.

Beta-Sitosterol - A phytosterol found in Goji berries, it is used to treat sexual impotence and prostate gland enlargement.

Betaine - A substance found In Goji berries which is used by the liver to produce choline, a compound that calms nervousness, enhances memory, promotes muscle growth, and protects against fatty liver disease.

Betacyanin - The red color in beets and red prickly pears, it has anti-oxidant power with cancer and tumor fighting capability.

Caffeic Acid - A substance found in cucumbers that reduces swelling when the cut cucumber is put on the skin.

Carminative - Any substance that reduces gas formation in the intestines.

Carnosine - This is a substance found in muscle meats and is made from the two amino acids beta-alanine and histidine. It is an anti-oxidant and opposes glycation, a cause of aging. Although it is not found in any form of vegetable, the fact that it is found in beef muscle means that the body can make it from the amino acids.

Celiac Disease - See Gluten.

Chondroitin Sulfate - It is a substance, isolated from cattle or pig ear, consisting of sugar molecules bound together, and a deficiency of it in the body is one of the factors causing arthritis. For supplementation only pharmaceutical grade is recommended, as its composition varies depending on what source it comes from. In Europe it is a prescription drug for arthritis.

Chymopapain - See Papain.

Collagen - This is the substance that skin, tendons, arteries, cartilage and bone, yes bone is made out of. The body needs protein to make it. It also needs vitamin C to make it. It is destroyed by an enzyme called MMP. Inflammation involves excessive MMP activity.

Coumarins - These are found in celery and enhance the activity of white blood cells improving immune response.

COX Enzymes - Or Cyclo-Oxygenase Enzymes. These are enzymes that make inflammatory and anti-inflammatory compounds in the body. COX-1 enzymes make anti-inflammatory compounds (arthritis preventative) and COX-2 make inflammatory compounds (causes arthritis) from Omega fatty acids in our diet. Pain reliever pills work by suppressing the COX-2 enzyme. Unfortunately they also suppress the good COX-1 enzyme so while you take painkillers joint damage continues in the body.

CRON - Stands for Caloric Restriction With Optimal Nutrition. Excess calories in the diet has been found to be one of the causes of accelerated aging, and less calories is associated with less aging. High Glucose levels from high carbohydrate intake has been found to be very damaging to the body. See Glycation.

Cruciferous vegetables - These are all vegetables in the cabbage family, and can range from mustard to watercress. Known for their anti-cancer qualities, but not too beneficial for persons with low thyroid performance, with the exception of watercress and sauerkraut.

Cryptoxanthin - A form of vitamin A found in papayas.

Curcumin - The principle polyphenol in the spice turmeric. Scientists have found that curcumin has potential for treating cystic fibrosis.

Cyanidin - Anthocyanidins found in raspberries and contribute to their anti-oxidant, anti-cancer activity.

Cyperone - Found in Goji berries, it is of benefit to the heart and blood pressure.

Cysteine - An amino acid produced in the body from the digestion of the protein in meat, dairy, and fish. It is used by the body to make glutathione, a major anti-oxidant in the body. It's vegetable sources are oats and wheat germ.

Cystic Fibrosis - A disease caused by difficulty in the body for producing mucus resulting in inflammation of lungs, and difficulty in breathing. See Curcumin.

Cytokines - Hormone-like substances that can increase or decrease inflammation in the body. Excess inflammation is associated with arthritis, cancer, and heart disease. Inflammatory or anti-inflammatory cytokines can be promoted by the particular diet we have.

DHA - Stands for docosahexaenoic acid and is an omega-3 fatty acid that occurs in fish oil.

DPA - Stands for docosapentaenoic acid and is an omega-3 fatty acid that occurs in fish oil.

Diverticulitis - Small, protruding sacs of the inner lining of the intestine (diverticulosis) can develop in any part of the intestine. This occurs more often after the age of 40. When they become inflamed, the condition is known as diverticulitis. Diverticulitis is very common. It is found in more than half of Americans over age 60. Diverticulitis is caused by inflammation, or (sometimes) a small tear in a diverticulum. If the tear is large, stool in the colon can spill into the abdominal cavity, causing an infection (abscess) or inflammation in the abdomen. Risk factors for diverticulosis are a low-fiber diet. There are natural substances that can increase intestinal contractions and help clean out the intestines. See Chapter 6.

Ellagic Acid - research suggests that red raspberries may have cancer protective properties. The biggest contribution to raspberries' antioxidant activity are polyphenols called ellagitannins, a compound almost exclusive to the raspberry, which are reported to have anti-cancer anti-aging activity. Ellagitannins form ellagic acid in the body.

Ellagitannins - See Ellagic Acid.

EPA - Stands for Eicosapentaenoic acid and is an omega-3 fatty acid that occurs in fish oil.

Flavonoids - See anthocyanidin.

Flavonone - Another word for Flavonoid, see flavonoids.

Gingerols - Substances found in ginger that kill cancer cells.

GLA - Gamma-linoleic acid, an omega-6 fatty acid that occurs in vegetable oils.

Gliadin - See Gluten.

Glucosamine - It is a substance that can be made by treating crabshells and shellfish shells with acid. The body converts it to glycosaminoglycans which is a component of cartilage, the hard smooth substance inside our joints and connecting tissues. One of the authors used it with success to restore cartilage to normal. It is generally warned by manufacturers that those with shellfish allergies should not use it but the allergens are in the flesh of the shellfish not the shells so it is not likely that pure glucosamine has much allergen in it. It is claimed that many studies have shown no benefit from it for arthritis but when these studies where examined by Dr Raymond Schep, he found that those studies included the use of "NSAID" painkillers. These would counteract the effect of the glucosamine.

Glucosinolates - These are compounds stored in cruciferous vegetables. The plant also stores myrosinase in its cells When the plant is chewed by animals the glucosinolate is mixed with the enzyme myrosinase to release isothiocyanates which has a sharp burning taste, thereby discouraging the animal from eating much of the plant. However, these isothiocyanates (see sulforaphane) have powerful anti-cancer properties.

Glutamin - See Glutathione.

Gluten - A protein that occurs in wheat, barley, and rye. It is made of gliadin and glutenin. Some people are allergic to the gliadin and severe allergy can cause celiac disease, an inflammation of the intestines.

Glutathione - It is the major anti-oxidant in the body. Anti-oxidants have been shown to counteract cancer and heart disease. It is made in the body and is a "tripeptide" which means it is made of three amino acids, cysteine, glutamine and glycine. Amino acids are derived from protein in our diet. Whey protein, parsley and rooibos tea have been shown to increase glutathione levels in our body.

Glutathione Peroxidase - This is an enzyme that destroys lipid peroxides, a chemical name for rancid fat in the body. Rancid fat increase the level of free radicals in our body associated with increased levels of heart disease and cancer. It contains selenium, a trace element we get from nuts and seafood, with Brazil nuts being the one of the foods with high levels of selenium.

Glycation - This is a process by which glucose bonds to protein in the body damaging it and increasing free radicals and inflammation in the body. This leads to accelerated aging. (See CRON). Highlevels of carbohydrates (starches and sugars) in the diet increase glucose levels and increase glycation. The change from Paleolithic diet to Neolithic diet has increased glycation.

Goitrogens - Substances that lessen thyroid gland activity resulting in sluggishness, cold feet and morning lethargy. Cruciferous vegetables have some goitrogenic activity and although they are great cancer fighters they may not be good for people with low thyroid. Fluoride intake appears to be one of the causes of low thyroid activity. LOW thyroid is properly defined as a TSH test value that is HIGHER than the average value, not sky high as some doctors require.

Heterocyclic Aromatic Amines - These are char forming chemicals made when meat is exposed to excess heat and are considered to be carcinogenic.

HGH - Human Growth Hormone, see Secretagogue.

Hydrogenated Oil - This is the process of reacting hydrogen with vegetable oils to make them harder and immune to rancidity such as the butter substitute margarine. This destroys the nutritional value of the oil as all omega fatty acids are destroyed.

Hydrogenated oil is not recommended for consumption as it is a non-natural substance that cannot be used by the body.

Isothiocyanates - See Sulforaphane.

Kombu - See MSG, Umami.

Krill Oil - Oil made from krill, a small animal that occurs in vast numbers in the ocean. Blue whales, the biggest mammal on earth, feed on these. A perfect source of Omega-3 fatty acids

LA - Stands for linoleic acid and is a omega-6 fatty acid that occurs in vegetable oils.

Lentinan - A compound found in mushrooms that empowers white blood cells to destroy cancer cells.

L-Ergothionine - A compound found in mushrooms that strengthens the liver and lessens cataract formation in the eyes. Highest in shitake mushrooms.

Limonene - A substance found in grapefruit that is a potent anti-carcinogen and that remains for up to 24 hours in the body, much longer than anti-oxidants from tea and chocolate.

Lipase - An enzyme that digest fats, breaking them down into fatty acids and glycerin.

Lutein - This is a carotenoid (plant form of vitamin A) that occurs in highest quantity with zeaxanthin in kale and then also in high quantity in spinach. They have been found to lessen the incidence of macular degeneration (which can end in blindness) especially in people over 65.

Lycopene - A potent anti-oxidant that occurs in tomatoes and even in higher amounts in watermelon. Considered to have anti- cancer and anti-prostate cancer action.

Lysyl Oxidase - This is an enzyme that forms elastin tissue in the skin, veins, arteries, and lungs using the amino acid lysine that we get from protein. It is a copper containing enzyme and when animal diets are low in copper death occurs from aneurysms and circulatory defects.

Macroautophagy - This is a process in which the body repairs itself after eating meals, and the body can only do this under fasting conditions. Digestion takes apart the food and can also be damaging to the body. This one of the reasons given why caloric restriction increases lifespan, See CRON.

Melatonin - A substance the helps sleep and is only produced by the body in darkness. Artificial light lowers the amount of melatonin in the body. It is also found in cherries.

MMP - Stands for matrix metalloproteinases. These are enzymes that destroy damaged collagen and cartilage in our bodies. If collagen and cartilage gets damaged faster than the body can replace it then arthritis and osteoporosis results. Vitamin C and glucosamine can accelerate the formation of collagen and cartilage and omega-3 fatty acids can reduce excessive MMP activity due to inflammation.

MSG - Monsodium Glutamate, flavoring agent. See Umami. Although MSG can be made synthetically, Kombu is by far a better source, as it also supplies iodine which tends to be deficient in our diets.

MSM - Abbreviation for Methyl Sulfonyl Methane. This is a sulfur containing substance that strengthens weakened tendons and ligaments.

Myrosinase - See glucosinolates.

Neolithic Diet - (See also Paleolithic Diet.) The eating of agricultural food, especially grains such as wheat, barley, corn, rice, oats, noodles, and pasta. Humans have only recently with the start of agriculture started eating this diet. It is of high calorie content. Even though it is our modern day diet it appears to be problematic, leading to diabetes and life shortening (see CRON.)

Neuroblastomas - Cancer cells in nerve tissue.

NSAID's - Non Steroidal Anti-Inflammatory Drugs. Synthetic drugs that treat the symptoms but not the cause of inflammation in the body and the joints and arthritis. The true cause of inflammation in the body is a lack of omega-3 and omega-9 fatty acids that we get from the right kind of oils in our diet. The body make anti-inflammatory hormones called cytokines from these.

Oleuropein - A polyphenol found in olive oil that inhibits both cancer and heart disease.

Omega-3 Fatty Acid - A compound found in oils of animal origin such as fish oil. It is reduces inflammation in the body that promotes arthritis, cancer and heart disease. The body can also make it from Alpha-linolenic acid which occurs in vegetable oils.

Omega-9 fatty Acid - A compound found in oils of animal origin such as fish oil. It reduces inflammation in the body that promotes arthritis, cancer and heart disease. The body can also make it from oleic acid which occurs in vegetable oils.

Omega-6 Fatty Acid - A compound found in oils of animal origin such as fish oil. It promotes inflammation in the body which in excess is associated with arthritis, cancer and heart disease.

Oncogene - A proto-oncogene is a normal gene in cells. Due to inflammation, or a lack of anti-oxidants, a proto-oncogene can be mutated into an oncogene. Oncogenes are found in cancer cells and prevent the death or destruction of the cancer cell, allowing it to survive and grow. In the cancer section of this book we discuss a study where omega-3 and omega-9 fatty acids reduce oncogene levels in cells but omega-6 fatty acid increases oncogene levels.

ORAC Value - This is a measure of the anti-oxidant capability of substances in other words its ability to destroy free radicals specifically the peroxyl or peroxide radical. It is thought that the higher the ORAC value, the greater the ability of the substance to combat cancer, heart disease, and inflammation. The compound trolox which is a water soluble form of vitamin E is used as a measuring stick, and the ORAC value reports how much trolox it would require to get the same anti-oxidant capability as the compound being tested. Ground Cloves has the highest value and limes are on the bottom of the list.

Paleolithic Diet - (See also Neolithic Diet). The eating of meat, fish, fowl, leaves, roots and fruits from the wild. This is a low calorie hunter gatherer diet, and the diet humans have been eating for millions of years. There are still some isolated tribes eating this diet and they have no heart disease, cancer, arthritis, or diabetes. It would be impossible for the majority of the population to follow this diet today but we can move to it somewhat by including as much as possible venison, caribou, wild caught seafood, and wild plants such as mustard, watercress, cranberries, mushrooms and berries in our diet .

Papain - Enzymes found in papaya that help in the digestion of protein.

Pain Relievers - See NSAID's.

PCB's - Stands for Polychlorinated Biphenyls. Used in electrical equipment and transformers it has polluted the environment and has been banned in the USA since 1979, but persists in sediments and water.

Pelargonidin - See Cyanidin.

Phagocytes - Also called white blood cells. These can pick up chemical signals from bacteria or damaged parts of the body, signaling them to go to that part of the body. They then engulf and destroy foreign particle, bacteria, and dead or dying cells. Vitamin C upregulates (empowers them) and glucose from sugar or starch downregulates them. Almost everybody has low white blood cell activity, resulting from excess blood sugar and vitamin C deficiency. Severe infection requires very high amounts of vitamin C to empower the white blood cells to generate enough hydrogen peroxide to destroy the infection.

Phosphatase - An enzyme found in milk that promotes the absorption of calcium by the stomach from the milk. This enzyme is not found in pasteurized milk; here the term milk means unpasteurized milk. It is also popularly called "raw" milk but there is no reason for this name, do they call pasteurized milk cooked milk? We don't call cucumbers raw cucumbers. Pasteurization of milk destroys the phosphatase enzyme leading to mal-absorption of calcium. Proper "raw" milk is becoming increasingly difficult to get. Maybe we should outfox the "pasteurized' milk crowd and call uncooked milk certified milk, a form of milk that mammals have been consuming ever since they were invented.

Physalin - A substance found in Goji Berries that helps in combatting leukemia.

Phytosterols - Cholesterol like substances found in plants. Sesame seed has highest phytosterol content known. Evidence suggests that the phytosterol content of the diet is associated with a reduction in common cancers. Phytosterols affect host systems potentially enabling more robust antitumor responses, including the boosting of immune recognition of cancer, and influencing hormonal dependent growth of endocrine tumors. In addition, phytosterols have effects that directly inhibit tumor growth, including the slowing of cell cycle progression, the induction of apoptosis, and the inhibition of tumor metastasis.

Phthalides - These are found in celery and lower blood pressure by relaxing arteries.

Polycyclic Aromatic Hydrocarbons - These compounds are formed when meat is heated to very high temperatures by barbecuing, grilling and frying. It is not found in meat that is heated to the boiling point of water at 100° C or 212° F. It is recommended that meat be grilled at as low a temperature as possible. These compounds have been shown to increase superoxide radicals in the body, and persons consuming the most amounts of barbecued meats have been shown to have higher rates of cancer. Properly and carefully cooked meat though, is an excellent food and contains the anticancer substance carnosine, and the cysteine in meat proteins promotes the manufacture of the anti-oxidant glutathione in the body.

Prostaglandins - Substances made by the body from fatty acids. The body uses omega-3 fatty acids to make series 3 prostaglandins which are anti-inflammatory. The body uses omega-6 fatty acids to make series 2 prostaglandins from omega-6 fatty acids which are inflammatory. Excess inflammation is associated with most disease, especially cancer, arthritis and heart disease.

Prostatectomy - Surgical removal of the prostate gland usually done when it appears cancerous. This will not address the true cause of cancer, which is a lack of anti-oxidants in the body.

Protease - An enzyme that digests protein by splitting it up into amino acids, or building blocks of protein. See also MMP.

Protease Inhibitor - Protease is an enzyme that breaks down and digest protein in the body. The protease inhibitor inhibits the digestion of protein. In the hunter gatherer diet beans were never eaten because they were inedible. (Paleolithic diet). This is due to the protease inhibitor that the bean makes to protect itself from being eaten. Then it was discovered that the cooking of the beans destroyed the inhibitor and made them edible. (Neolithic diet) . However this increased the calorie load and a less healthy diet.

Protozoa - Tiny animals and plant like animals found in water and can be seen with an ordinary microscope. They can cause disease in humans with poor immune system capability.

Proxeronine - It is found in pineapples but is much more concentrated in Noni Juice. The body makes xeronine from it, a substance that signals cells in our body how to repair themselves and how to function properly.

Quercetin - See Rutin.

Rutin - An anti-oxidants found in buckwheat, amongst other they inhibit platelet aggregation and strengthen capillaries.

Schizophrenia - A mental disorder. Also found in some persons that have gluten allergy or celiac disease.

Scurvy - A deficiency of vitamin C in the diet resulting in immunodeficiency , brittle bones and tooth loss It is popularly thought that this only affected sailors in the middle ages that were months at sea, but in actuality most people show some affects of scurvy if they have no resistance to colds and flu, or tooth abscesses, or osteoporosis.

Secretagogue - A substance that causes the body to secrete something. The term is mostly used for a formulation of nutrients specifically designed to increase the production of Human Growth Hormone (HGH) in the body. HGH declines with age and this decline is regarded as one of the causes of aging.

Sex Hormone Binding Globulin - Or SHBG. This is a protein that can bind to testosterone and make it unavailable to the body. Persons with low testosterone levels age faster and have less energy . Oats extract and nettle root extract can prevent the binding of testosterone to SHBG, resulting in higher testosterone levels and feeling younger, more alert and stronger.

Silicon - What sand is mostly made out of. Plants can absorb silicon, especially cucumbers and barley (beer) and provide it in usable form to the body for skin and bone health.

Silymarin - A substance found in thistle plants such as milk thistle and artichokes that can protect the liver against toxins, and that can also heal damaged liver tissue.

Solavetivone - It is found in Goji berries, and is a powerful anti-fungal and anti-bacterial compound.

Sulforaphane - A strong anticancer substance found in cruciferous vegetables. This is only released by cutting or chewing the vegetables, which releases the enzyme myrosinase that forms sulforaphane. It is in a family of chemicals called isothiocyanates. Other isothiocyanates are also released by cruciferous vegetables. The enzyme can be destroyed by cooking. Broccoli has been found to have the highest amount of sulforaphane but all cruciferous vegetable contain it.

Testosterone - This is a hormone made in the body. It is called a male hormone but females make just as much of it as males, except in females most of it is converted to estrogen. It is responsible for hair growth, muscle mass, and bone mass. It is now thought that aging is caused to a large extent by decline in these hormones. Although supplements of mainly artificial forms are controlled by doctors there are natural plant materials that can stimulate higher levels such as Suma, Oat extract (Avena Sativa) and Nettle root.

Theobromine - This is a substance found in chocolate that is similar to caffeine from tea and coffee but not quite as strong. It gives feelings of well being and is a stimulant.

Thromboxane A2 - It is a substance in the body that promotes clumping of platelets (red blood cells) which is blamed for causing stroke. Cinnamon has powerful anti-oxidants in it that suppress thromboxane A2.

Transfats - These are fats where the molecule gets bent out of shape, which can be caused by partial hydrogenation, and then the molecule can no longer be utilized by the body. It must be disposed of by the body as waste. Cis shape: at left (boat, normal) Trans shape: at right (chair, abnormal). Consider, if you purchase some item such as bicycle etc in a kit that has to be assembled. If one part is put in the wrong way the whole assembly will malfunction. Likewise the body has to have all the correctly shaped molecules to build and run the body.

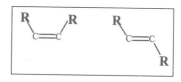

TSH Test - A test for thyroid stimulating hormone. The higher the test value is, the lower the thyroid function.

Tocopherol - The chemical name for vitamin E. There are 8 forms of vitamin E that occur in nature; alpha, beta, gamma and delta tocopherol, and alpha, beta, gamma and delta tocotrienol. Our government only recognizes one form of vitamin E, namely alpha tocopherol, and claims it is the only form used by the body, but in actuality all forms have been found to have some affect on the body. Red palm oil is a good source of the tocotrienols.

Tyrosine - Tyrosine is an amino acid that the body uses to synthesize proteins and thyroid hormone. It occurs in meat, fish, milk and eggs. Kelp has iodinated tyrosine particularly suited for the thyroid gland. Vegetable sources of tyrosine are mustard, carob and soybeans.

Umami - A taste that can be experienced by taste buds in addition to sweet, sour, salty and bitter, and is best described as savory. Kombu made from kelp has strong savory flavor. Kombu is a natural source of glutamate.

Ventricular Repolarization - The period of time it takes the heart to recharge after it beats, so it can beat again. It was found that eating carefully cooked fish or scallops lessens the time needed by the heart to repolarize.

Xeronine - See proxeronine.

Zeaxanthin - See Lutein.

About the Authors

Currently, Dr. Schep is the chief chemist for Colonial Dames Company, a cancer and nutrition consultant for Dr. Paul Savage of Chicago and a consultant for specialist health, nutrition and anti-aging with top anti-aging researchers in the world. Dr. Schep has also worked for the UCLA School of Public Health, studied natural medicine through a correspondence course at Bastyr University and he has lectured on animal nutrition at the University of Hawaii.

Upon completion of doctorate degrees in chemistry at the University of Pretoria, South Africa, Dr. Schep engaged in diversified fields of research and development for many years. With this extensive experience and knowledge, he has been involved in developing new ways to incorporate natural ingredients into cosmetics. Dr. Schep has dedicated his scientific research and findings to the development of the effective treatment, Rolenta. He is highly respected for his research, development and technical support in the fields of cosmetics.

Dr. Schep has worked in close contact with Dr Paul Savage who almost single handedly created the American Academy of Anti-Aging Medicine, and Dr. Savage has consulted with Dr. Schep on a several occasions. See http://www.worldhealth.net/pdf/Tips_Antiaging.PDF. His main area of interest is replacing synthetic drugs with superior natural cures.

Nicole Kellar-Munoz is an Operations Support Specialist with the Federal Judiciary and was a legal assistant and paralegal for five years before beginning with the Federal Judiciary in 2004.

From the age of 10, Nicole has been a working part of her parent's natural bath, body and home-care manufacturing companies in production, manufacturing, and packaging, and specialized in sales, marketing, and training. She also has been a ghostwriter for several educational textbooks on business, training, and marketing for Turn the Rock Publishing and co-wrote "Quick-Fix Healthy Mix", a guide to creating healthy, filling meals quickly, easily and on a budget.

Using the principals in this book, Nicole has lost over 60 pounds and has become passionate about distance race walking, successfully participating in multiple relay races and, this summer, completing her first half-marathon.

Nicole is determined to provide a healthy and green home and it is a joy for her to pass down to her son the knowledge, skills, and health consciousness her family and co-author, Dr. Raymond Schep, have passed down to her. Nicole lives with her husband, son, and dog in Scappoose, Oregon.

Following are Dr. Schep's Organizations and Accomplishments:

- Recognized by the Men and Women of American Science
- Member of Society of Cosmetic Chemists
- Member of the Scientific Advisory Committee for the Cosmetic, Toiletry and Fragrance Association
- Ten scientific publications in international journals
- Retains 10 United States patents

Presently Dr. Schep is testing anti-aging discoveries by playing Lock in the second team for the premium Belmont Shore Rugby Club at age 63. The club is, at present, number one in super-league standings of all U.S. rugby clubs nationwide. Player ages range from 22 to 35. In order to do this, he had to cure his arthritis. He found natural cures work the best, and he had to overcome aging with bioidentical hormones and super foods.

Other Fine Books from F+W Media

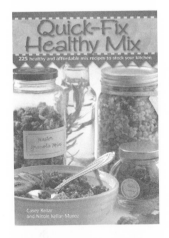

QUICK FIX, HEALTHY MIX

Stop over-paying for foods loaded with toxins, unhealthy fats and sugars. Instead, make your own high-quality mixes at a fraction of the cost. Quick Fix Healthy Mix has more than 225 easy-to-make recipes, made of easy-to-find, eco-friendly ingredients. Casey Kellar is the author of six books on living in a natural lifestyle and has consulted with small food companies to help them with their formulas.
ISBN 13: 978-1-4402-0385-5
softcover - 240 pages - Z5032

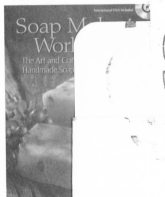

THE SOAPMAKER'S WORKSHOP

...e pure cleanliness and ...nd-crafted soap This ...alks you through the ...instructions for using ...ting up a safe work- ...ye and oils. You'll also ...how to make liquid ...es.

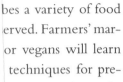
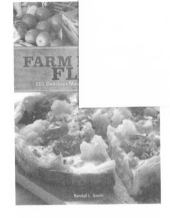

...bes a variety of food ...erved. Farmers' mar- ...or vegans will learn ...techniques for preparing the food, and why farm fresh food is a better choice for healthy eating. Author Randall L. Smith is Executive Chef at the iconic Clocktower Resort in Rockford, IL.
ISBN 13: 978-1-4402-1397-7
softcover - 304 pages - Z9166

Visit our website at www.betterwaybooks.com